SPARTAN STRENGTH

Your complete guide to building serious strength for life

BY JACK LOVETT

IronLife

IronLife

SPARTAN STRENGTH

BY JACK LOVETT

Editor	**Jon Lipsey**
Editorial Director	**Joe Warner**
Managing Editor	**Chris Miller**
Designer	**Ian Ferguson**
Photography	**Glen Burrows**
Additional Photography	**Victoria Kemp**

SPARTAN STRENGTH ISBN **978-1-9998728-4-7**

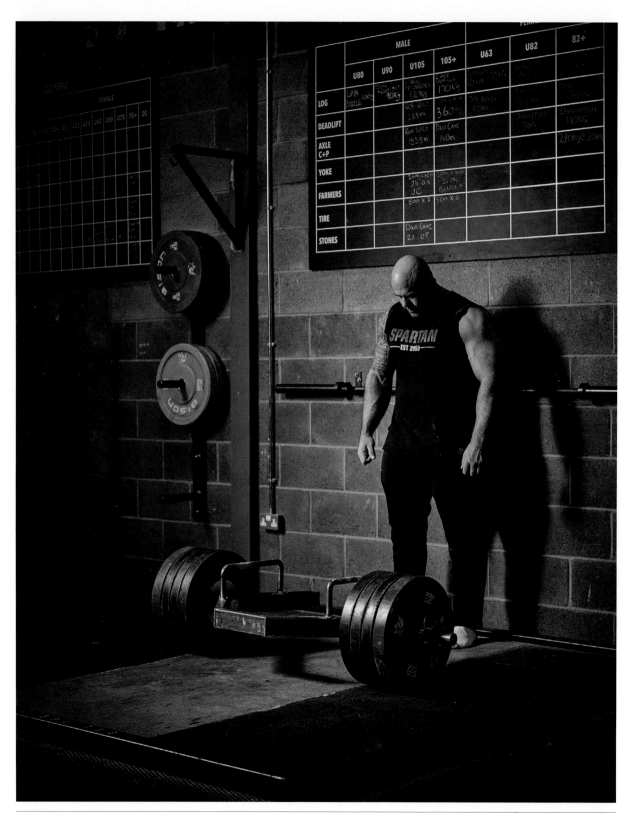

ACKNOWLEDGEMENTS

While I'm comfortable putting my own name to the methods and ideas in this book, I'd be remiss not to acknowledge the inspiration I have taken from various coaching authorities in my pursuit of knowledge. In particular: Joe DeFranco, Christian Thibaudeau, Louie Simmons, Jim Wendler, John Meadows and Stuart McGill. My library is full of their work and I will always be grateful.

Theory is one thing, but it's in the application that I have learned my most valuable lessons. In that regard I'd like to thank every single client I have had the good fortune to work with over the years. All the wins, losses, successes and mistakes have enabled me to be where I am today. They will continue to define me in the future too.

Without the support of my team at the Spartan Performance gym in Consett, I would not preside over such a successful training environment. This truly is a team effort. To Laura, Jenny and (not so little) Jack, I thank you in ways I don't express enough.

Finally to my editor and the true driving force behind Spartan Strength, Jon Lipsey. Little did I know a chance meeting at a seminar back in 2013 would lead to this. Your support and guidance throughout have been invaluable and appreciated.

I TAN I EPI TAS

DONNA MOORE WORLD'S STRONGEST WOMAN CHAMPION

'I'm 100% confident that Jack can help you get stronger'

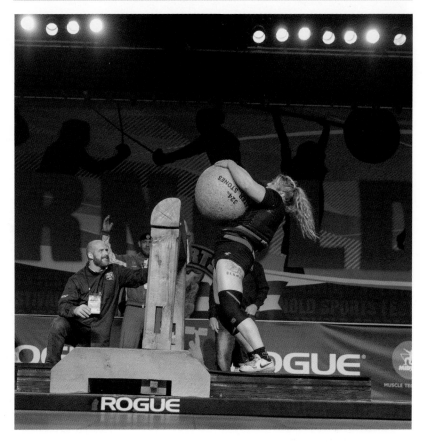

I've trained with Jack Lovett for years now and it's always a positive and educational experience. I always bring my best every time I train with him and I'd never go unprepared because he is always the same with me. He knows exactly what we're trying to accomplish in each session.

I'm 100% confident that if you're reading his book, Jack can help you get stronger. And I'm 100% confident that he can make improvements to anybody who follows his strength training system, as long as you're willing to put in the effort. If you're focused and determined and want to work, that's the key. You can't just turn up half-hearted. If you're willing to put the work in, Jack will complement everything you do and make you a better athlete.

Through working with Jack I've gained a better understanding of everything I'm doing and what I'm trying to achieve. It's all about progress and if something doesn't go as planned Jack always finds a way to address it and fix it. We'll assess why things happened and we'll discuss it too – he'll tell me why he thinks it happened, I'll tell him why I think it happened, and by the next time we met we'll have a solution.

When I'm preparing for an event I like to be coached only by Jack because of the mindset that it gets me in, which is that if there's a task to achieve then we're just doing it . That's the end of it. I've been to three World's Strongest Woman competitions and three Arnold World Strongman championships with input

from Jack and I've won the worlds twice. I broke the Atlas stone world record at the Arnold as a result of the time we spent training Atlas stones. All of Jack's cues and drills, I just hear them in my head. It's an automatic thing. I just hear his voice. I'd say all my Atlas stone world records have been down to the work I've done with Jack.

When I started training with Jack I had an idea about how to train but he just makes the skillset better. He brings all the elements that I might not see – he refines it all and puts it together to create a stronger package. We're always working on technique. If you can't get that right then you're not going to get anywhere. I couldn't have done any of my recent competitions without his coaching involvement.

Whenever we start a session, Jack will always ask me how I am and find out what has been going well and what hasn't. Then he outlines what he wants us to achieve in the session and the targets that we're aiming for. What I really

like is his ability to modify the session as we go to suit my needs on the day.

When you work with Jack it's always educational. You'll learn something from every session. You can ask him anything and he knows the answer. But he also empowers you as an athlete to think about how you can make yourself better, and that has really helped my mindset. As long as you show the right desire, he's 100% dedicated to your cause.

MEET THE EXPERT

Donna Moore was World's Strongest Woman champion in 2016 and 2017, as well as runner-up in 2018. She is also a two-time Arnold Pro Strongwoman champion, a two-time Arnold Amateur world champion and a Rogue Record Breaker Atlas stone world record holder.

TOM HAMILTON
POWERLIFTING CHAMPION

'Books like this are so important – a resource like this is gold'

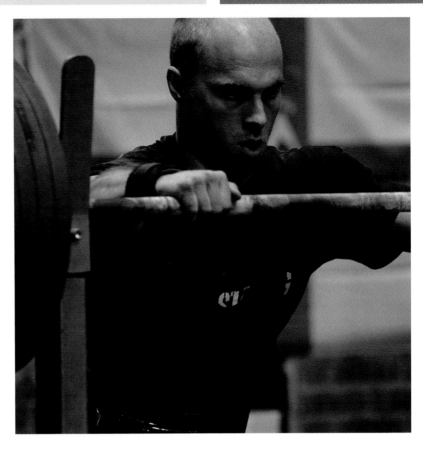

In the six or seven years I've been training with Jack, his approach has helped me improve my lifting numbers and win powerlifting competitions. I work with Jack because I have a lot of respect for him as a person as well as a coach. He's straight-talking and I like that. He doesn't sugar-coat stuff or beat around the bush. It's straightforward advice that works. But at the same time he's very supportive and very encouraging. He gives you information which is going to have impact. He has competed as an athlete himself and I find that inspiring. He walks the walk.

Usually in competition I'm pretty confident and I back myself, but I remember one time when I'd had a break from competing in powerlifting for a while and I was getting back into competition. I was putting pressure on myself and trying to compare my efforts with my previous performances. I had a bad training session when I missed a target and I was like, 'This competition is not going to go well'. But Jack was so supportive and encouraging. He helped me to get my head around it and rationalise it properly, and when it came to the competition he had filled me with confidence. I went on to hit personal bests in a couple of lifts, which I wasn't expecting.

One of the biggest things I've taken from working with Jack is that doing the basics really well is where people should invest their training time. Everyone could benefit from getting stronger and having good movement quality, and that's what Jack's approach is about – doing things in the right way, focusing on quality. This will help you in every area of life, whether that's in the gym, on the sports field or in your overall health.

I've learned a lot from him that I now use when I'm coaching. He has so much knowledge and so many skills that he's able to wear many different coaching hats. He has got such a deep well of knowledge that he can tap into and I'm always really impressed with his variety of tools, all based around solid principles, for getting the job done.

I'm lucky that as well as being coached by Jack I've also watched him coach a lot. I feel like he understands me and knows how to push me in training to get the most out of me. But I've also seen him tap into different aspects of his personality and his coaching abilities to cater to different people, which is a great skill and one that I really admire in him.

I think books like this are so important. There's loads of information out there and for the uneducated person – in a fitness sense – it can be easy to get sucked in to following bad information or the wrong people. So a resource like this is gold, really. It'll stand the test of time as well, which I always think is a great indicator of quality. It's all built on solid foundations and proven methods, and it's about doing the basics well. Focusing on those things is going to do so much more for you than hopping from one training fad to another.

MEET THE EXPERT

Tom Hamilton is a coach at W10 Performance in London and head of education at the International Fitness Business Alliance (IFBA). He was World Drug Free powerlifting champion and Overall Best Lifter in 2016, British Drug Free powerlifting runner-up in 2016 and UK Drug Free Bodybuilding runner-up in 2014.

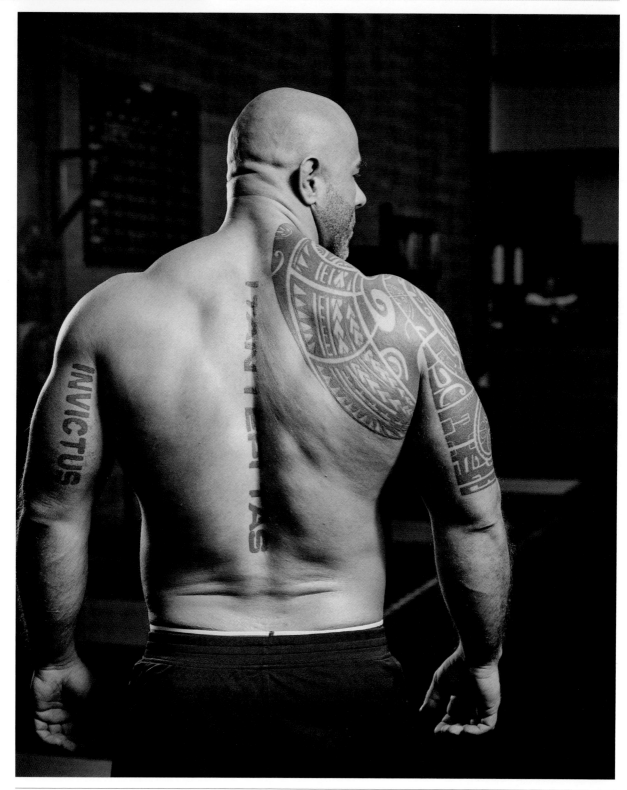

Harness the Spartan spirit to build real strength

You might be wondering why this book is called Spartan Strength. The short answer is because my training business (which has nothing to do with the film *300*) is called Spartan Performance and we specialise in getting people stronger.

I chose that name for my training business, and the gym I now run in the northeast of England because I've always been fascinated by Sparta, the ancient city-state whose citizens dedicated their lives to training and excellence. True, their efforts were centred on getting prepared for conflict but I see no reason why their focus and work ethic can't be applied to our own everyday battles, whether that's entering a strongman competition or just being the best version of yourself that you possibly can be.

STRONG START

This book is for anyone who wants to maximise their strength training potential, whether you're a regular gym-goer or a personal trainer looking for inspiration and guidance on how to help your clients excel. It's not an exhaustive treatment of my strength training knowledge and experience. It's a distillation of everything I have learned since I first picked up a barbell, and it contains the essential information that I believe you need to get seriously strong. This has been forged during the thousands of hours I've spent coaching clients, ranging from World's Strongest Woman champion Donna Moore to gym newbies who are just starting out on their strength training journey.

The manual you're holding is a reflection of what I believe matters most if you want to get stronger. I'm not trying to impress you. I'm not trying to entertain you with fancy exercise variations you've never seen before. I'm giving you what works. That's why the structure of the book – which starts with the foundation exercises that I want you to master before you start loading up the bar and ends with an overview of programme design – is designed to make it as accessible and as effective as possible.

JUST REWARDS

I wanted to do this because I know how rewarding strength training can be. It has given me so much – including the discipline to achieve my goals and the mental toughness to push on when faced with a challenge – and I want to pass that on. One of the things that I love about strength training is that it doesn't discriminate. It doesn't matter whether you're a complete beginner or a World's Strongest Man competitor. If you apply yourself in the right way with the right effort, you'll be rewarded.

There's a phrase my warrior heroes used before going into battle and I've adopted it as the Spartan Performance motto. It resonates so deeply within me that I have it tattooed down my back. It reads 'I TAN I EPI TAS' and it basically translates as 'with it or on it'. Simply put, you either return victorious from battle with your shield, or you return on it, having given everything to the cause. That's the mindset I use to approach every session, and it's one that I'd encourage you to adopt.

Yours in strength,
Jack Lovett

CONTENTS

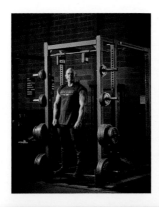
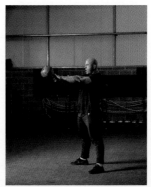
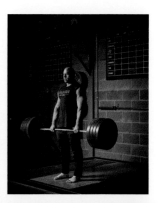

INTRODUCTION	01 FOUNDATION MOVEMENTS	02 KEY LIFTS
014	**026**	**058**
Discover the training philosophy that underpins this book and defines the Spartan Strength approach	The better you get at these foundation movements, the greater your potential to get bigger and stronger	These big bang-for-your-buck lifts will be the cornerstone of your training for your entire lifting career

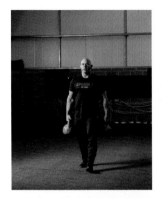
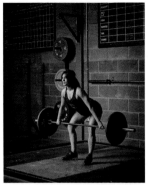
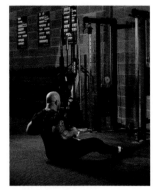
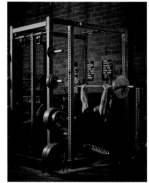

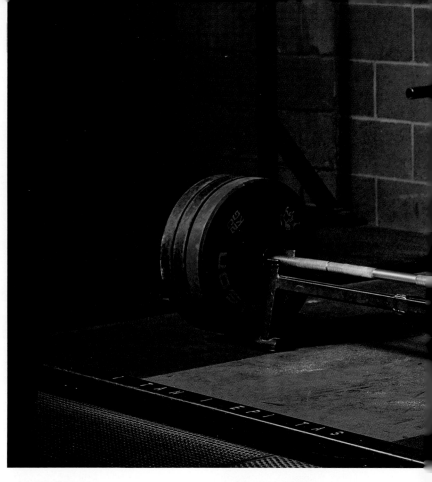

Why strength training matters

Here's why I think you made the right choice in picking up this book and why getting stronger will help you hit any goal

1 IT'S NEVER A WEAKNESS

This is something I believe to the bottom of my very soul. In all the years I've been in the industry, I've never come across someone who is *too* strong. If you can get stronger, that's going to improve you. It's the cornerstone of my programmes and my gym ethos.

You can strength-train successfully without needing to be a powerlifter or a competitive athlete. Regardless of your goal, it's going to improve things. If you want to improve endurance, get stronger and your endurance will improve. If you want to build more muscle mass, a stronger muscle has a greater potential to be a bigger muscle. If you want to be more powerful, if you want better definition, if you want better density of muscle – there is no downside to pursuing strength training.

That's something I like to get across because when some people think of strength training they think you're trying to go out and set new world records. That's not the case at all.

2 IT REQUIRES PATIENCE AND DISCIPLINE

Progressing at strength training requires a period of years. It's not a quality that can manifest overnight and then suddenly you're where you need to be. It's a skill that you have to practise and hone again and again. And ultimately, the improvements will come through patience and through discipline. That's the minimum that's required.

That doesn't always work well, especially with young guys. They come and see me and they want everything yesterday. But it just doesn't happen that way. Those who stick to it, however, develop patience and discipline – and those are qualities that, in my opinion, are essential for success in all aspects of life. What you do in the weight room can transcend the walls of the gym.

3 IT BUILDS MENTAL STRENGTH AND RESILIENCE

Someone who is new to strength training will get newbie gains. And they're fantastic, aren't they? But they sure don't last. You might go from an 80kg deadlift to 100kg, 120kg, 140kg, 160kg, 180kg... and then you might start to stagnate.

Newbie gains come very easily because of the initial exposure to a new training stimulus. But they're not sustainable. If you stay in the game long enough you're going to end up toiling away for what probably seems like marginal gains. Some days you'll feel great, most days you'll feel OK and the rest of the time you'll feel like shit. To be successful in this endeavour, irrespective of goal – whether you want to be world's strongest man or just strong for life – you have to keep going.

More than just patience and discipline, you've also got to have mental strength. It's a mental battle, not just a physical battle.

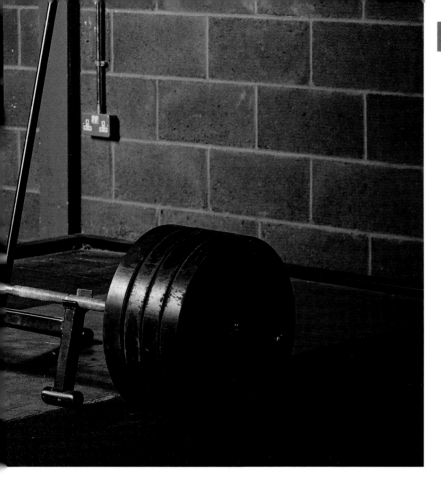

My plan for success

There's a question I ask myself before I start any strength training plan, and it's one that I'd pose to any client: how badly do you want it? That's something that you've got to be honest about. Because if I want it badly enough then I will put in the work that's required.

The next thing I ask is, what are the things that are required? I don't find it stressful or too much pressure to have a challenge put in front of me because I know the systems that I need to put into play and I take a lot of inner strength from that. So it's pretty simple. If I have a target in mind, I'll write a programme starting at the finishing date and working back to where I am. I'll put a smart, structured and progressive training programme in place. And I know that if I follow that correctly then I will improve.

I also like to be in command of as many variables as possible. Those variables are training, nutrition and recovery. I have a direct impact on these things. I can't do anything about my genetics – I can't change my height, for example – but I can have a positive impact on everything else. Granted, some people have greater natural aptitude for strength than others. Some people are naturally lean. Some people are born bastards and look lovely from the start. But that doesn't mean that you can't improve.

4 IT'S REWARDING

There is nowhere to hide in a weight room. If you've got 100kg on that barbell, that's 100kg that you've got to move. It's not something that you can cheat. It's not something that you can fluke. You've got to be prepared physically, mentally and from a recovery perspective and, ultimately, you have to perform. But I don't want that to seem like a negative thing.

I find it very motivating. Very inspiring. Because the achievement that you get is all yours. If you take your deadlift from 140kg to 141kg, I don't care if someone else lifts 450kg in competition – you've made progress and nobody can take that away from you. That's what I try to instil in my athletes and my clients. Don't worry about the struggle – and it is going to be a struggle – because nothing in this life worth having comes easy.

5 IT DOESN'T DISCRIMINATE

Most people assume my gym is called Spartan Performance because the film *300* came out and the actors in that all looked fucking amazing. Well, not quite, though it certainly didn't hinder business in the early days! I actually called it Spartan Performance because during my studies of Ancient History, Latin and Greek at University I did a dissertation on the Spartans. And in ancient Sparta, physical culture was a massive component of their lifestyle. The women and men trained together – it wasn't like the guys were the only ones exposed to physical training. And that's been my philosophy since day one; training does not discriminate in terms of age, ability or sex. If you learn how to train smartly and you implement strength training methods astutely, then you will gain appreciable levels of results.

Meet the man behind Spartan Strength

Jack Lovett, coach, author and strongman champion, talks to Spartan Strength editor Jon Lipsey about his will to win, what drives him as a coach and why he will never accept less than 100% effort

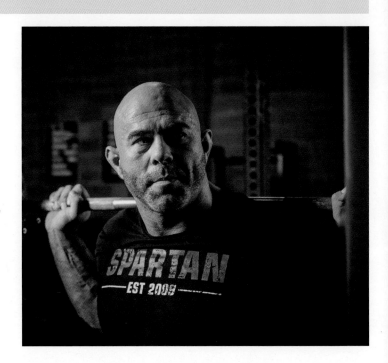

What makes you different as a coach?

If you ask me what separates me from other coaches, I don't really know! Maybe my clients could answer more objectively. But what I do know is that I'm constantly communicating with leading coaches and authorities to identify more effective methods and systems. I'm fascinated by anyone who delivers results and in learning directly from them I hope to emulate the success they have had with their clients using such methods.

I am also happy to freely acknowledge my limits. My methods are certainly not the only way to achieve results. There may be many other methods to achieve the kind of results that I'm talking about. But there's a very specific reason why I haven't included them in the book – it's because I don't use them. As a coach and educator it is my responsibility to ensure I deal specifically in methods I have used and got results with. I could cheat and pass someone else's opinions off as my own. But I'm not about to become a charlatan to sound smarter. I'm only going to speak definitively on exercises that I have found to be incredibly effective year in, year out.

Why have you selected the exercises in this book?

I've focused on exercises that have provided me with the biggest bang for my buck over my training lifetime. They've provided the biggest return not only for my clients, but for my business too. My business only succeeds if people keep getting results, making progress and coming back.

These exercises have provided the greatest return to the people who have come through my door – and now

the readers of this book can learn those same movement patterns, exercises, loading parameters, sets and reps that have been effective in my facility with my clientele under my coaching and in my environment. These exercises have been at the core of all programming at Spartan and been constantly refined through years of 'in the trenches' coaching.

A key point to note is that I may not use all of the exercises included with all of my clients all of the time. They are simply tools in a very large toolkit and, as a coach, it's crucial that I choose the right exercise for each individual. Why? Because everyone is different. For example, take a high-end athlete – I'll give you the three I am most proud of working with: UFC legend Ian Freeman, professional footballer Alex Gilliead and two-time World's Strongest Woman Donna Moore. Even combined, they don't all use every exercise that I have described in this book because how they train is based upon a needs analysis. For every client I ask myself the same question: how can I best achieve the results for my client with the tools from my toolkit?

What do you remember about your Britain's Natural Strongest Man victories?

The first year, in 2009, was very easy. That's no disrespect to the athletes I competed against. It just worked out that way. It was the first time that there was a British Natural Strongman competition and you had some great competitors in there such as Ben France and Phil Learney, but I think won it with a couple of events to go. Everything just seemed to go my way. That's the thing about strongman competitions

– you can have 10 people competing and if you change just one event you can get a different result on the podium. It happened to be that the events suited me. I enjoyed the entire experience and I can't say that it was a massive challenge.

But in 2010 there was a competitor called Ben Kelsey, who is one of the best strength athletes I've ever come across. When I beat him there was a huge amount of relief and a huge amount of satisfaction.

What made him the best athlete you had come across?
I consider him to be a good friend so I'm not going to kiss his arse too much. I believe his head may be big enough already! But there is no denying he is a phenomenal athlete and competitor. He has been my biggest rival throughout my career on the competition scene. He managed to get to the televised World's Strongest Man finals in 2014 weighing all of about 18 stone [114kg], which is tiny by WSM standards. He has few weaknesses and has given me a hiding many times. So to beat him made it a very worthy win. In 2009 I won by about 15 points but in 2010 I won by half a point. And it was a victory that I'm very proud of.

What's the difference between achieving something as an athlete and as a coach?
I consider myself to be an athlete first and foremost. I've competed in sport from a young age. And it was always about winning, whatever sport it was. When I built Spartan Performance it was actually for somewhat selfish reasons. Nowhere had the type of gym that I wanted to train at. I'd been over to Joe DeFranco's in the US and nothing could compare in the UK, so I built one myself.

Achieving things as an athlete was essential to me, and I think that's integral to who I am as a coach. Even though I have made mistakes, I've always been 100% supportive to any client I've ever worked with because when I work with them, their goal becomes my goal. You know, it's hard to put into words the satisfaction that I felt when I saw Donna Moore run riot at World's Strongest Woman in 2017 and then go to the Arnolds the following year and do so all over again. It was as satisfying as the win I had over Ben Kelsey in 2010.

What drives you as an athlete and a coach?
I'm driven to be the best I possibly can be, and in turn I'm driven to help my clients become just that too – the best they can become. I have a great deal of difficulty relating to people who are not wiling to give their all in the pursuit of a goal. That's not to say that I belittle a goal because you don't want to become World's Strongest Man. That's nonsense. But if you say you want something and I give you the answer as to how you can achieve it, it's difficult for me to understand if you don't do it.

Maybe that's the athlete, the competitor, inside of me, but whenever I've had a competitive goal it's simple. I want to run *this* fast or lift *this* much weight, so I break it down to work out what I need to do to achieve that goal. Then I'll commit everything to achieving it. Maybe that's a good thing.

> ## 'I'm driven to be the best I possibly can be, and in turn I'm driven to help my clients become just that too – the best they can become'

Maybe that has limitations for me as a coach. I don't know. I just don't understand half efforts. If someone comes to me and wants 100% of the result but is only willing to put 40% effort in then there's going to be an awkward silence.

How hard is it to get strong?
At the end of the day, what we do isn't magic. Adding 20kg to your deadlift or another realistic goal is not a miraculous occurrence. I'm not talking about becoming proficient in seven languages in one week! My job is to get someone to be stronger or more muscular, to have better body composition or to improve sporting performance. It's not a gamble. What I do works.

There are proven methods and proven systems to increase strength or add muscle mass. Granted, genetics come into play and some people will build strength or muscle more easily. Some people will burn fat more easily. But the point is, if you want to get stronger, you can. If you want to build more muscle, you can. If you want to drop body fat, you can. Why? Because I will show you a system that is proven to be effective. And not only has it been proven to be effective over the past 10 years but I'm constantly educating myself, researching the subjects, trying to find a better, more efficient way.

I don't need a pat on the back for getting somebody stronger because, in reality, it's not that fucking hard. When somebody comes with a goal, we break it down logically for them so that it is system-based with a good support network. Then they need to have the desire within themselves to be consistent. I don't think that's asking too much.

Get Spartan strong

These are the ideas that underpin the way I train, and the way I want all my clients to approach their own training. These concepts support the fundamental principles behind this book, so if you apply them to the best of your ability I guarantee you'll see positive results

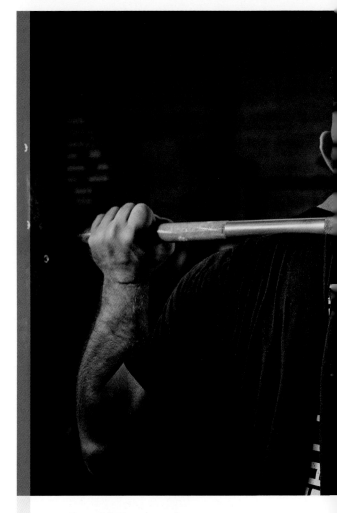

SPARTAN STRENGTH LESSON #1

Solid foundations lead to lifting excellence

I like to instil good habits from day one with all of my clients. What exactly does that mean? It means that they lift with perfect form. I want them to understand what the movement is that we're going to perform, why we're doing it and how to perform it optimally.

Anyone going on a training journey needs to build that solid foundation of discipline because it's empowering. I want someone to graduate from my foundation lifts so that they understand not only how to do an exercise but why we do it – like why we perform a Russian kettlebell swing rather than an American kettlebell swing. It's empowering because when they progress to the barbell lifts, they'll not only have technical ability but also a positive mindset. If an individual has a lot of flaws in their exercise technique, they won't be able to perform the moves effectively. So they won't enjoy what they're doing and they'll soon lose that positive mindset. You get people who shy away from deadlifting or squatting heavy because they don't have the skillset to perform those exercises correctly. And when the session gets challenging, they crumble.

The better you come out of the foundation chapter in this book, the more you milk the advice there for all it's worth, the better everything else is going to be down the line. Because when we ultimately get to the barbell lifts, there's not much

Real life results

When everything is in your favour, it's easy to be positive. But in real life things are rarely set up in a way that's ideal and allows you to feel 100% positive about your outcome. Let's take a typical day for me as an example.

I'm writing this at 8.30am, but this isn't the start of my day – I've been coaching since 5am. And as soon as I finish working on this book I'm coaching through to 1pm. Then I've got a two-hour gap where I've got to squeeze in a big deadlift session before seeing more clients and meetings into the evening.

I need to make that deadlift session as productive as possible so I ask myself, how badly do I want it? How focused will I be? I'm busy and tired, but will I let it affect my session or will I make sure that this session is a success? That decision is down to me.

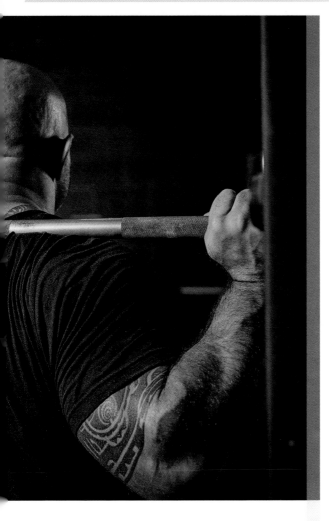

I also have a friend here training with me, and we went out to eat last night so I didn't get as much sleep as I ordinarily would. When I woke up this morning I didn't want to get up. But I had a simple choice. What was I willing to do today to get the most out of my session? I could set the tone before my session started – take command of the day, in whatever circumstances I find myself in, or let it get on top of me. So I set my alarm early to make sure I could eat a decent breakfast.

Is today optimal for me? No. But in reality, apart from professional athletes, I don't know anybody that has an optimal day. I always know I'm following a structured programme, so what's on my schedule today is attainable. It may be more challenging in some capacity than the previous session that I did. But it's not impossible.

else to add. We can come up with some crazy shit but it's not half as effective as certain people who are all over social media would suggest. There's no point in racing to get someone to the barbell back squat if it means they have poor technique when they get there, because where do they go from there?

Performing the foundation section properly will also enable you to build the mental discipline required to get strong. In other words, the discipline to leave the ego at the door. The discipline to listen to the coach – or, if you're coaching yourself, the discipline to read the cues that we espouse in this book and put them into practice.

TAKEAWAY TIP

The Foundation Movements chapter (which starts on p26) is the most important section of this book for two reasons. First, it'll teach you the movement patterns that will underpin every exercise you perform for the rest of your training life. And second, if you approach it in the right way, you'll adopt an attitude to lifting that will help you to maximise your strength training potential. It really is that important.

SPARTAN STRENGTH LESSON #2

Chase perfection for maximum return

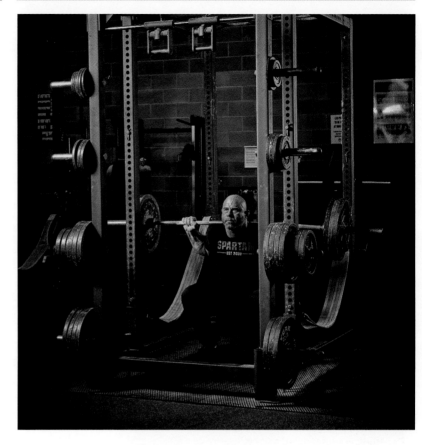

My philosophy at Spartan Performance is that, from the first second you come through the door, everything you do must be perfect. Every pedal on the bike, every mobility drill, every jump and every throw. I want it all to be perfect. Why? Because I am determined to get every client the maximum return possible from every single session.

Remember, I'm playing the long game here. Let's say you come in and I have you begin with some foam rolling. Beneficial, sure, but hardly the most exciting thing on earth, so it's quite easy to drift off and just go through the motions. In reality that's not going to ruin your session immediately. But what that means is that you are not fully engaged. You are not fully focused and you are not fully committed.

Why is that important? Well, at the beginning of a session, if your application isn't a 10 out of 10, if your buy-in to the exercise isn't a 10 out of 10, that's going to have a cost somewhere down the line. And I take that seriously.

BE THE BEST
One thing I tell my staff, inspired by something the coach and mentor Alwyn Cosgrove said, is that we need to be the best part of our clients' day, every day. I don't care what's happening in our personal lives – we blow the mind of the client every time. We're on top of every single

rep. It's my belief that positivity breeds success and leads to more positivity. Conversely, if you do something sloppy or sub-par, you might not have a disaster within that session but it can spread like a disease and cause issues down the line.

If you're a coach and you're seeing quite a few movements where your client is just not engaged or buying into it, it may be that you need to change the movements. Or it may be that you need to coach them better. Every aspect of a coaching session is an opportunity to get more out of a client and unless you've got an insanely motivated professional athlete and everything in their life is just rosy coming into the session, then your clients will be coming in with some issue or some baggage. Even then, they still want to get a kick-ass session.

TIME AND AGAIN
Every coach has to remember that the time they have with their clients

comes at a premium and you want to make sure that every single second of every session counts. So yes, every rep counts, and yes, every rest period counts. Everything you do within that session should be aimed at making the session as productive as possible.

If I'm doing my job right, every one of my clients is going to leave the session better in some regard than when they walked in through the door.

TAKEAWAY TIP
You don't only make an effort when you're doing a heavy rep or an 'exciting' exercise. I want every single thing you do in every single session to be of the highest quality possible. A drop in standards in anything you do in the gym will ultimately erode your overall strength training potential.

SPARTAN STRENGTH LESSON #3

Develop an iron mind to build an iron body

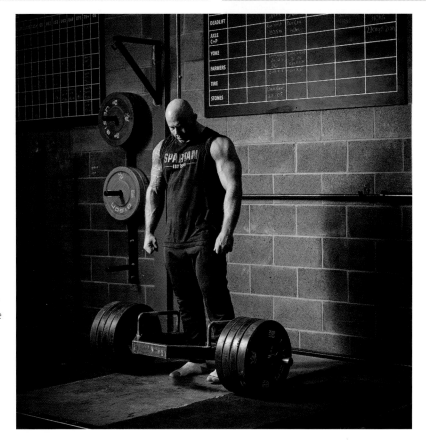

If you build discipline by graduating from the foundation chapter in this book then you're going to be able to approach sessions with greater focus and mental toughness. So when the sessions and the exercises get tougher, you've got the discipline in your mind and the discipline in the technique to get through it. If you take that path then I'd say that you're automatically in the top 20% of trainees I've ever encountered.

Once you're in that top 20% and you've got the focus and the discipline, how can you get even more out of a session? For me it comes down to this: how badly do you want your result? How badly do you want to achieve the goal? Once you've answered that question you can get more specific and ask yourself this: what are you willing to do to achieve that goal?

TRAIN SMART AND HARD

The vast majority of people who I have encountered throughout my coaching career simply do not train hard enough every session – set to set, exercise to exercise – to elicit a change and a result. Strength training does not discriminate, everyone can get stronger, but it's not a case of just turning up and doing the sets and reps and getting the result. Unfortunately, it doesn't work like that. You have to fight, on every single set and every single rep. You've got to force that adaptation. You've got to force that result.

And you know what's even worse? The better you get and the more training time you have under your belt, the harder you've got to work for fewer gains. When you start out you get the newbie gains but eventually they run out. So someone like me has to put in a monumental effort to see my main lifts go up by even a few kilos over 12 weeks. That's why you need mental strength and fortitude to do what it takes.

YOU'RE IN CONTROL

To make each rep as good as it can be, I have the attitude that I move the weights, the weights don't move me. So when I take the bar out of the rack for a squat, I have the mental discipline to brace before I begin the descent. Then I lower under control. If I'm performing loaded carries of 60-80 metres and my forearms are on fire and all common sense tells me to put the weights down, I ask myself, 'How badly do I want the result?' If I drop them because my forearms are burning, the weight is dictating what's happening. I put them down when I'm good and ready. That's the only approach that's ever delivered any semblance of success for me.

It's about taking ownership of the training session and of your life. We're in control of everything in the gym and that's empowering. And if you make the right choices, when it was easier to make the wrong choices, guess what – it's going to motivate you.

TAKEAWAY TIP

If you want to get seriously strong then the thing you need to focus on strengthening first is your mind. If that's resilient, you'll always be able to dig in when the going gets tough – and I can promise that it will get tough – so you can extract as much as possible out of every rep. A strong mind makes a strong body.

How to keep a training diary

Accountability is key to sustained progress in the gym –and keeping a training diary increases your accountability in every single session. It means you come to the gym with a plan in place, so you know what's required and stand a far greater chance of getting it done

HARD DATA
As a coach, the more information I have, the better the job I can do. Even if you're not working with a coach, keeping a training diary means you have specific information that is invaluable in progressing session to session. You want to know every set, every rep, every weight and every rest period – the specifics of what you're doing in each session. That way, if you're missing weights that you know you should be getting but you can see your plan was appropriate, what's the deal? You know there's something to address. It could be a technique flaw or that your recovery has been sub-par. These may be simple examples but my point is clear. The more information you have to hand, the better you can identify a weak link or why something is breaking down – and fix it.

COMPLETE PICTURE
In theory, if you're programming correctly, there should be no missed reps. But in reality you will miss reps from time to time, so I also like to track how the individual is feeling. What was the energy level like going into the session? What was the motivation level like going into the session? What was the recovery like from the previous session? If the training diary says you've done the right sets, reps, rest and weight but something's not right, then you can look for the other bits of information. You may realise that when you came into the session you had four out of 10 for energy levels, or that your hamstrings were stiff from the previous deadlifting session, creating a negative carryover for squatting. That kind of information will illuminate flaws in recovery, sleep or nutrition.

PRACTICAL USE
I assess the data for every single session that I'm working together with a client. Before they come in, I'll familiarise myself with their previous performances. Then when they come into the gym we'll have a brief conversation so I can find out what I'm dealing with in terms of energy levels and recovery. If you're training yourself, you can still track your previous performances and you can also be introspective. You can analyse yourself to work out the condition you're in when you start the session. The only thing I'd say is that you've got to be careful not to become too analytical because that can take away from the session itself.

PERFORMANCE MARKERS
I track key performance indicators (KPIs). If you have a 12-week training programme, we'll choose key indicator exercises pertinent to your specific goals. I might give you a five-rep max in the key lifts – squat, deadlift, bench press and military press. But I also want my clients to have a good level of relative bodyweight strength, so I might also track your press-ups and pull-ups by getting you to do max pull-ups in one go or max press-ups in 60 seconds. Those lifts will all appear throughout the programme so you will be able to assess your progress in them without having to do extra assessment sessions. I've found that if you re-test too many times during a 12-week period, progress can stagnate. For that reason, I like to test at the start and end of a 12-week programme.

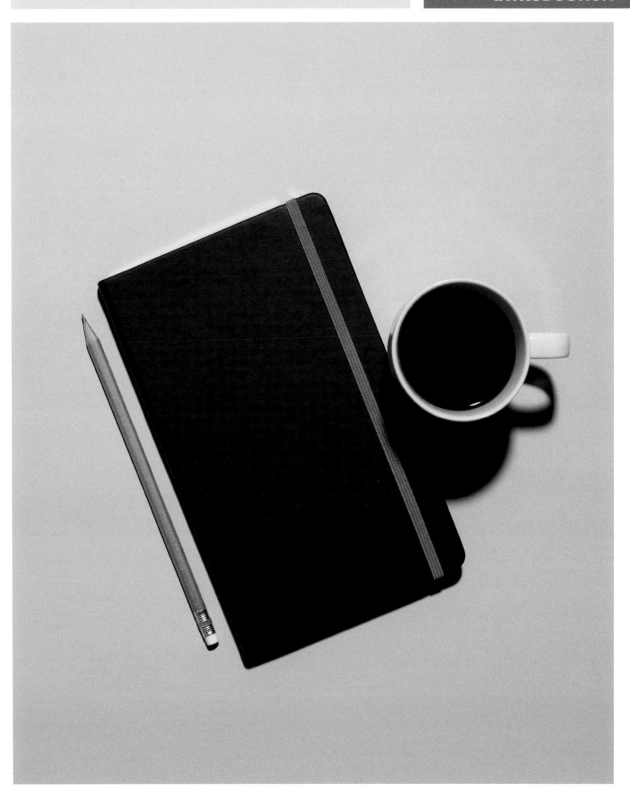

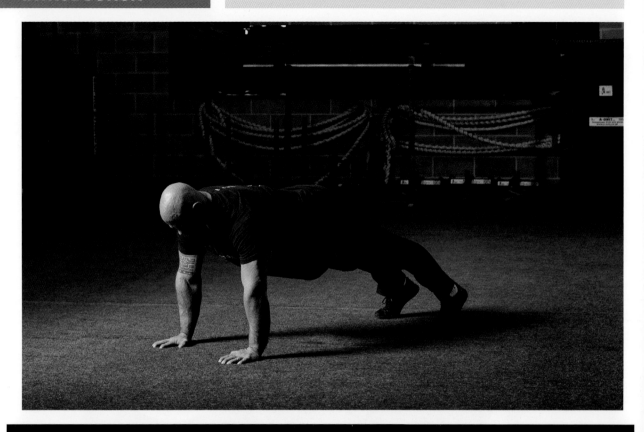

How to use this book

Here are the main chapters in the book and
how they fit together

01 FOUNDATION MOVEMENTS

02 KEY LIFTS

I've tried to make this book as easy to follow as possible. Your first task is to work your way through the exercises in chapter one, Foundation Movements, until you can execute them with flawless technique. From there I want you to build up an appreciable level of strength by using the key lifts in chapter two. The moves outlined in the following three chapters will complement your core strength training work and help to eliminate weaknesses.

The exercises in this book don't comprise an exhaustive list of useful moves but they're the ones I believe will give you the biggest bang for your strength training buck. Once you've got to grips with them you'll be in a position to apply the information in the final chapter and start to build your own strength training programmes.

I cannot emphasise this enough – the set of exercises in this section are the most important collection of moves you will ever perform. How competent you are in these lifts will determine your strength training potential. If you skip this section or move on with flaws in your technique, you will be limiting your potential to develop strength further down the line.

The lifts in this chapter are the ones that should form the backbone of your programmes for the rest of your strength training career. They are the most efficient moves and the ones that will allow you to get seriously strong. You can use these lifts for life, so you should always be looking to refine and improve your technique.

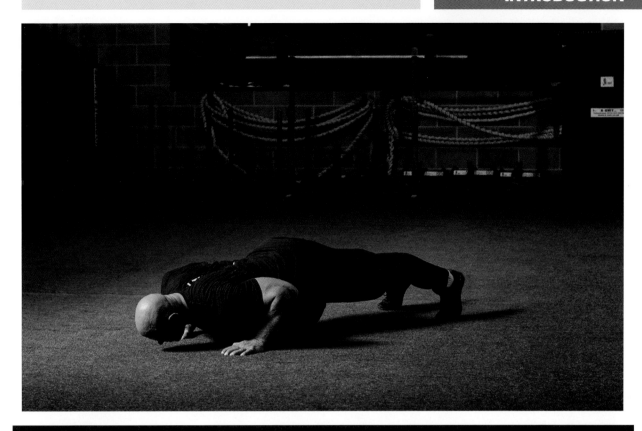

**03
LOADED
CARRIES**

**04
POWER
TRAINING**

**05
HYPERTROPHY
EXERCISES**

**06
PROGRAMME
DESIGN**

This chapter goes into the many benefits of loaded carries in detail. In short, they are an excellent tool for building strength, stability and an iron mind. It's rare that a simple and accessible exercise such as the farmer's walk is so rewarding in terms of strength benefits. That's why I love them and why I want you to milk the moves in this chapter for everything they're worth.

Power training is vital to anyone who wants to get stronger. First, you can use these moves to ignite your central nervous system and maximise the potential of your training session. Second, you can use them to increase your rate of force development, which will have a positive carryover to your ability to shift heavy weights. This chapter contains the key power moves I want you to focus on.

You might wonder what hypertrophy-style exercises are doing in a strength book and the answer is simple: a bigger muscle has a greater potential to be a stronger muscle. But I don't just want you to lift for show. All the exercises in this section have been selected because they are excellent assistance exercises that will help you to iron out any weaknesses in your key lifts.

In this chapter we bring together all the exercises and concepts we've covered in the rest of the book and give you an overview of how I would typically use them to structure a training session. I also outline how I would begin to build a progressive and periodised training plan so that you can take charge of your own strength training journey.

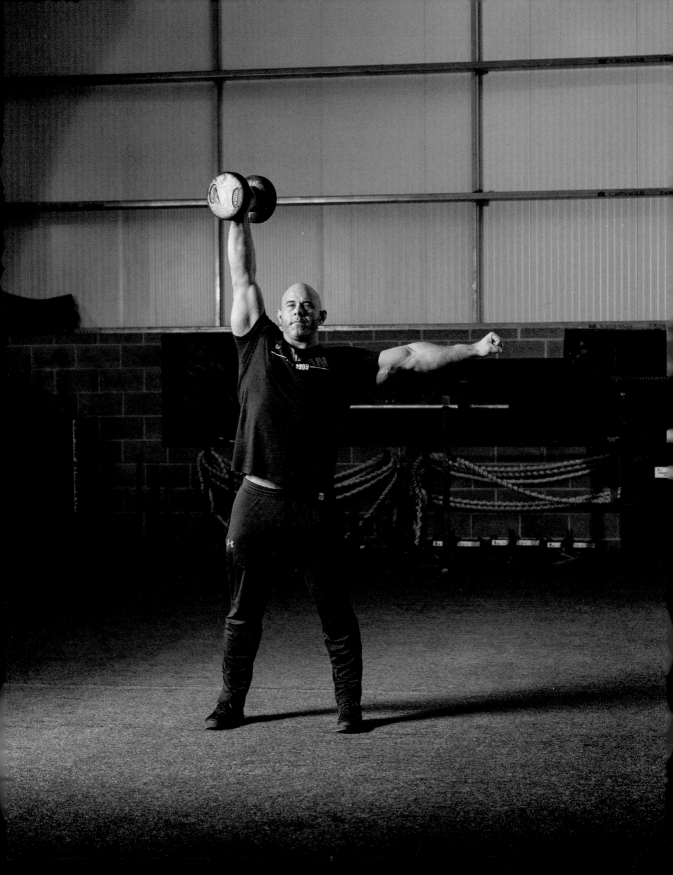

01.

FOUNDATION MOVEMENTS

You might expect that every exercise in a strength training book is about loading as much weight onto the bar as you possibly can. Sure, that's our end goal. But the best way to achieve that goal, in my view, is to follow what I consider to be the most effective system for long-term progress. It's one I have refined over 20 years of strength training and coaching. And that system, regardless of who you are, starts with mastering some fundamental movement patterns.

There are probably pretty good ways of building strength that don't involve doing all of these moves. But I'm not looking for 'pretty good', I'm looking for the optimal way, and this is the best method I've found to prepare people to get the most out of subsequent heavy barbell training.

My approach is about seeing the bigger picture. If you develop technical mastery of these foundation lifts then that will give you the perfect platform to start your strength training journey. And it is a journey. It's not a shortcut or a quick fix. It's a game for life. So it's vital that you build a solid base.

Over the years I've seen many people move on to the barbell lifts too soon. They might be doing half-decent weights on the bench press, but they are poor at the bodyweight variations of that movement such as the press-up – and those bodyweight versions are enormously beneficial. Not just in terms of chest development but also for core strength, for shoulder health and even just for teaching an individual how to move their elbows correctly.

If you skip the moves in this section, which many people who don't train with me tend to do, then you'll leave yourself with weaknesses that may not come to the fore immediately but they will come back to haunt you down the line. You're going to have difficulty performing one of the main barbell lifts as well as you need to, and that issue is going to come down to a flaw within a fundamental movement. It makes no sense to me to try to fix something later that you could have easily avoided by doing things a bit smarter at the start.

I've noticed poor fundamental strength skills more and more since we've had a physio and sports therapy component to the gym. We have many patients who train elsewhere who all exhibit the same issues, such as shoulder pain thanks to a lack of upper back development and lower back issues thanks to not knowing how to brace, and maintain a brace, throughout heavier lifts. While the moves in this section aren't a cure-all for any injury, mastering these movements and their variations works well to address weaknesses and develop muscular balance from the outset.

MOVES THAT MATTER

I've chosen the lifts in this section because I've identified key movement patterns that I want my clients to excel in. Each movement pattern has a base variation that can either be progressed or regressed according to you or your client's abilities. If we take the bodyweight squat as an example, a regression might be a squat using a suspension training device such as a TRX, and a progression would be a goblet squat with a dumbbell or kettlebell. Foundational movements are easily scalable, with multiple variations to match different levels of ability.

I want you to perform these lifts well but also to be able to perform them in relatively high volume too. That will help to build the base of strength, muscular endurance and work capacity that is vital if you want to go on to get seriously strong. There's a misconception with some of these exercises that they are somehow condescending to give someone – it's 'just' a press-up or

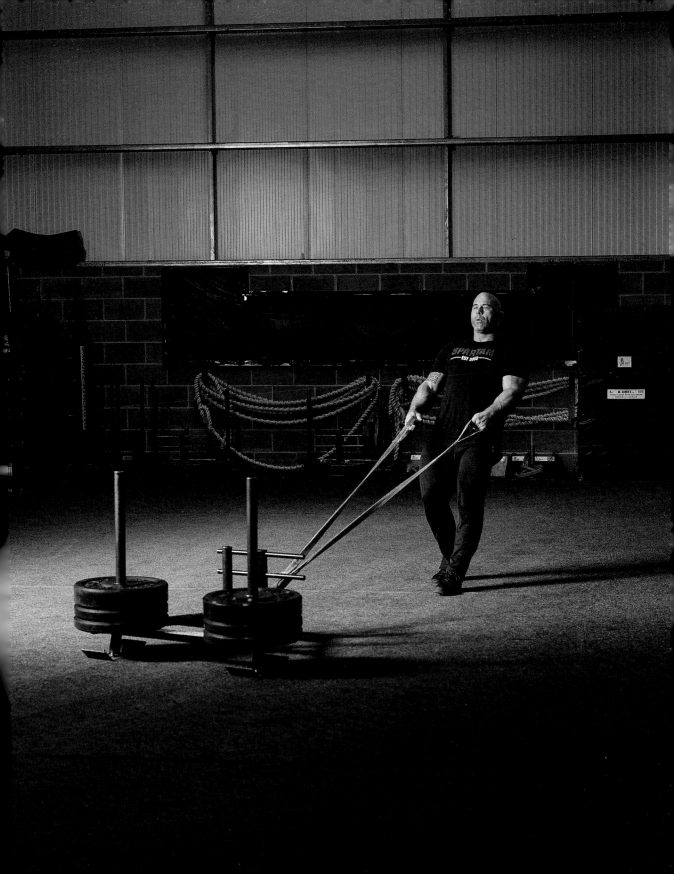

'It isn't just physical qualities that you're developing. The key quality for long-term success is discipline'

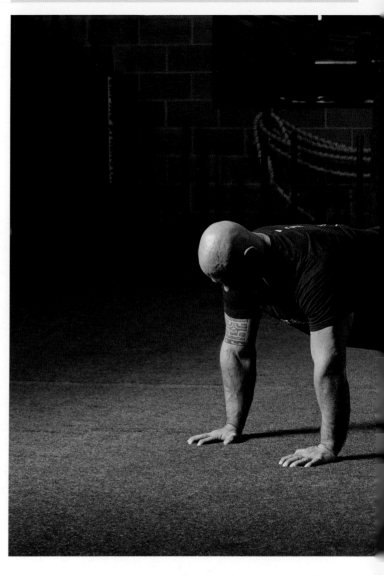

bodyweight squat, and therefore it's a glorified warm-up. I find it amusing that a lot of the people who have that view can't actually do the exercises properly.

Of course, if you're a coach, it can be a difficult concept to get across to some of your clients – especially younger guys. I understand that because when I was new to training, I was your typical adolescent who was easily distracted by the pictures and feats of strength relayed in the fitness magazines of the time. Trying to copy Mariusz Pudzianowski, who was winning World's Strongest Man by a country mile and looking like a superhero in the process, was far more appealing than spending time learning to retract my scapula. When Ronnie Coleman squatted 800lb [363kg] for two reps only weeks out from the Mr Olympia competition, you would have been hard pressed to convince me what I really needed to do was develop my goblet squat ability in order to lift better in the future.

Well, thank god I learned from my mistakes! All I can tell you is that anyone who assumes the exercises in this section aren't that challenging will soon come to respect them when they see and feel the effectiveness. It truly is about seeing the bigger picture and preparing your body and your mind in the most efficient and effective way possible.

DISCIPLINARY PROCEDURES
Crucially, it isn't just physical qualities that you're developing during this stage. The key quality for long-term success in strength training is instilling a level of discipline and learning to be consistent with it. Now, I'll freely admit that for some people, the fundamental movements are not the ones seen as the coolest or sexiest exercises. I accept that. But I'm looking for the optimal way to get the most out of barbell training, and this is what I've found that works.

The idea is that you learn the movement pattern so it becomes second nature. That prepares you so that, down the road, when we load you with weight on their back, the movement pattern is set so we don't have

to teach you that – we can worry about other things such as maintaining a brace and applying tension.

PREPARE FOR GREATNESS
I've seen again and again that these moves build the foundation from which you can progress to any goal. How well you perform the lifts later in this book will be dictated by the quality of the foundation you build at the start. If you get this bit right and maximise your potential in these fundamental movements, you'll find that you pick up other new techniques faster and, in the long run, you'll make better progress.

If you're looking for a real-world example, here's one that's hard to argue with. I recently hosted Dimitry Klokov, the weightlifting world champion and Olympic

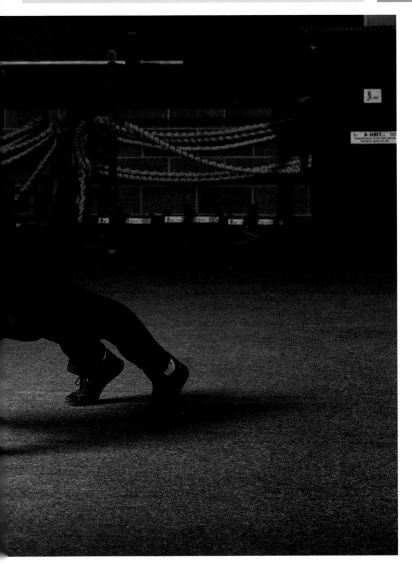

Takeaway tips

TECHNIQUE IS PARAMOUNT

The foundation movements aren't the most technically challenging exercises but I want you to understand the importance of executing an exercise optimally. Then I want you to execute it repeatedly until it becomes an ingrained movement pattern because how you perform a bodyweight squat when you graduate from the foundation section is the movement you'll use when you have a maximal load on your back. The hard work is done now. The better you come out of the foundation section, the better that will translate to success down the line.

DISCIPLINE GETS RESULTS

In my experience of thousands of hours of training clients, mastering technique instils discipline. It takes discipline to not just get the exercise technique optimised but also repeat it and to see the bigger picture. A lot of young guys in particular get very enthusiastic and as soon as they can do a few press-up reps they want to know how to do the next version of the press-up – and then the next and the next and it's a race to get to the sexiest-looking exercise. In my opinion, what they require is the discipline to focus on the basics and the exercises that will benefit them in the long term.

CONSISTENCY IS KEY

To excel and to graduate from this section in the fastest possible time and in the best possible way you need the appreciation of form, you need to master the form, you need the discipline to see the bigger picture – you may even need to regress yourself on certain movements – and you need the discipline to practice these movements and skills as frequently as possible. Because that's what they are – they're skills. The final part is consistency of application. You have to put in the work. You have to see it through. You have to do the thousands of repetitions.

silver medallist, at my gym to deliver some seminars. Everyone is in awe of the crazy lifts that he puts out on social media. The guy is an absolute freak. He's hands-down the most impressive strength athlete I have spent time with in person. And he's someone who started weightlifting later than his contemporaries and in his own words was 'slow and not very flexible'.

To remedy this, he spent an entire summer working not on weightlifting but on overall physical training: jogs, overhead kettlebell throws, handstand walking, press-ups, empty barbell lunges and a host of other moves. Foundation movements, in other words, and I'm willing to bet that he did countless sessions and reps in those movements. That's what built the foundation for him to go and be the incredible athlete that he is now.

> The better you get at foundation moves such as the press-up, the better equipped you'll be to add serious weight to big lifts, such as the bench press

Foundation lifts FAQ

I'm answering these questions in the exact same way I would answer them if I was asked them in my gym. It's not like I'm sitting here on a rocking chair reminiscing about 'back in the day'. Once I've finished writing these answers, I'm going to be back on the gym floor working with clients, putting my methods to the test.

I've been training for a while. Should I do other stuff while I work my way through the foundation lifts?

If you're a general-population client who is committed to training, I would convince you to see the bigger picture and stick to the foundation lifts. Maybe you are great at horizontal pressing but weak in other areas. If you're an athlete with a competition on the horizon then I'd do a needs analysis.

Even using the foundation lifts you can still satisfy an individual's hunger

to have frequent workouts – you can satisfy the need to feel like you've had a tough training session. A smart coach doesn't just make the client tired for the sake of it, but we do want to create a training stimulus and some clients associate feeling that training stimulus with progress. Well, don't worry – you can definitely get that stimulation with foundation movements. They can be incredibly challenging.

I'd also encourage you to have the patience to regress certain movements because this will benefit you in the long run. A client should be able to see that after just a week or so, but that comes down to coaching. I can write this stuff down on paper but you've got to get the client believing in you and believing in the process.

You can easily develop a full-body training routine that would differ every

day of the week just by using the exercises in this chapter. I could hit you with volume, with intensity or exercise variety. And crucially you are learning how to breathe, how to brace and how to maintain that brace. It's going to be a lot easier to learn how to do that while doing a press-up if you can already do press-ups, than it is by putting your maximal bench press on the bar and then teaching you how to breathe.

Can you build an appreciable level of physique using the foundational lifts? Absolutely. You can build muscle mass, you can improve strength and you can improve body composition as well.

How long should I spend on this section?

It depends on you and how hard you're prepared to work. I'd say between one and three months. If you're someone who has done all of the exercises in this section before, you may be able to perform them adequately, in which case it doesn't take a great deal of time for a coach to tweak their technique. It may feel like you're taking a step back but that's in order to take several steps forwards.

And if you have a decent training history it's not like these movements are going to kick your arse, which means you'll be able to add volume pretty quickly. For someone who is new to training, the process will take longer. At Spartan Performance the target we set ourselves is that – assuming the individual is injury-free and there are no limitations – we can take someone from zero training history to mastering the fundamental moves in three months.

How important is the load that I use?

I do have standards that I want you to reach but, along the way, my main focus is getting the most out of the

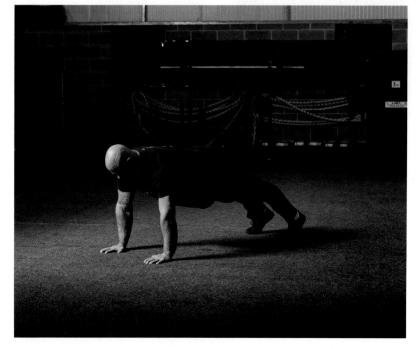

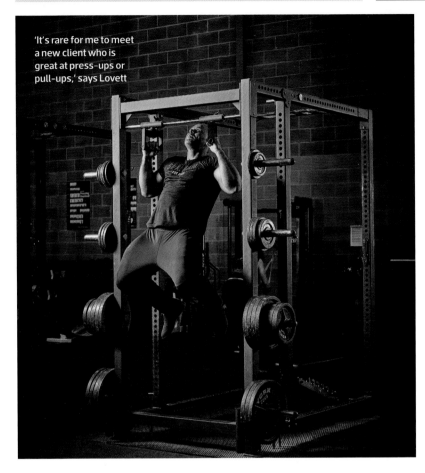

'It's rare for me to meet a new client who is great at press-ups or pull-ups,' says Lovett

least. So if you start goblet squatting with a 10kg dumbbell, instead of worrying about getting you to a 12kg or a 15kg dumbbell, I want to make sure that the 10kg dumbbell is giving us everything it possibly can. I want to milk it for all it's worth. Are you crushing it like it is 100kg? Are you bracing like it is 100kg? If you train like that you'll get a great workout with what, at face value, seems like a light load.

Ask yourself this – why does this foundation section exist? It's simple. I'm giving you these movements and telling you that if you do them in sufficient volume with the required technique, you will learn skills that are invaluable for, and can be immediately applied to, barbell lifting. At the same time you're building a foundation of strength and the work capacity and discipline that's going to serve you well down the line.

How do I know when I've become proficient in the foundation lifts?

I would advocate certain standards across the board. The first standard is the absolute confidence in knowing what a brace is, as well as being able to explain it, demonstrate it and maintain it. I don't care how many press-ups you can blast out if you can't perform and maintain a brace. After that I have certain requirements, whether that's reps to be achieved or loads to be used. The book will go into detail on that for each exercise in this chapter.

What should I do if I'm great at some of the moves and poor at others?

Everybody is going to have strengths and weaknesses. You may excel at bodyweight squats, in which case you go straight on to goblet squats. But maybe your press-up technique is

lacking and your horizontal pressing isn't great. That's fine because we can work on progressing or regressing those moves accordingly. With the goblet squat that's pretty easy – we just use more weight. And if you're struggling with press-ups then you'll stay on the bodyweight version with your feet on the floor until eventually you're able to progress that movement.

Nobody is going to be at the same level with every single movement. There is always something that they could perform better. For example, it's rare for me to meet a new client who comes through the door and is great at press-ups or pull-ups. They may struggle to get one press-up from the floor but they can easily get a variation of an inverted row.

How should I build the moves into a session?

You've got a couple of options. The most obvious are a movement-specific session and a full-body session. So you could focus on horizontal pushing on one day and horizontal pulling the next day. Or you could combine a horizontal push and pull in one day, squatting on another day and pushing and pulling vertically on another day, and then maybe perform hinge movement patterns the next day. One thing I do like to do is put core stimulus in every session.

How I break your sessions up depends on the individual. I look at their training experience and how many days a week they're training. If someone can only train three days a week, for example, I'd use a full-body split. Ultimately we want to put as much volume into these moves as possible. The more volume you can do now, the better it's going to serve you down the line.

Horizontal press

KEY MOVE PRESS-UP

TARGET
Men **15-20 reps**
Women **10-15 reps**
This isn't an upper limit – aim
for as many reps as possible.

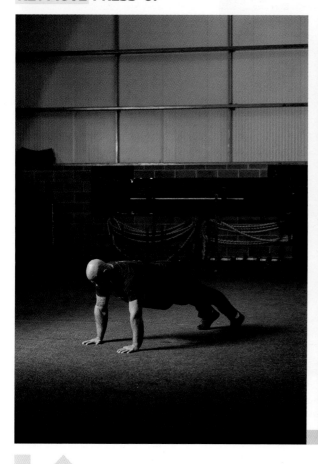

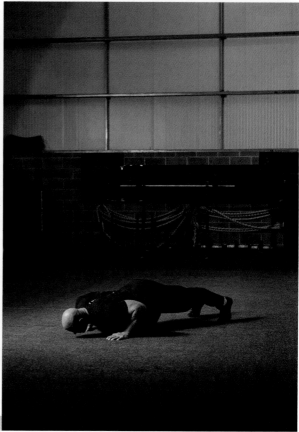

Everything I've ever done in coaching has led me to the firm belief that it's vital to develop a solid foundation in relative bodyweight strength before you progress to adding external load. The press-up and its variations are the best starting point for horizontal push training. Too many people ask, 'How much do you bench?' but that's really just the icing on the cake. What they should be asking is, 'How many press-ups can you perform?'

A press-up is the perfect preparation for progressing to a loaded bar later on. You'll also find that as your bodyweight ability increases, your body composition

will improve too. You also get good core stimulation and that's something that's often overlooked. Core strength shouldn't be an afterthought.

All foundational movements must be easily scalable to accommodate all levels of client. We therefore need suitable regressions and progressions. In the case of the horizontal press we can regress to a hands-elevated press-up or, if you need to progress the movement, adding external load via chains or using gymnastic rings. Whatever the client's level of experience, I always want to build great foundations before moving on.

PERFECT FORM

- Assume the press-up position with your hands and toes on the floor with your wrist, elbow and shoulder joints aligned.
- Engage your core and squeeze your glutes to raise your hips so that your body is straight from head to heels.
- Bend your elbows, keeping them close to your sides and not flared out, as you lower your chest towards the floor.
- Lower under control, pausing with tension across the shoulders and chest at the bottom.
- Press back up through your palms to straighten your arms and return to the start position.

COACHING MASTERCLASS

THE FLAW SOFT BODY

I see a lot of press-ups performed where there's no tension in the body and this often causes the individual to drop their hips, placing stress on the lower back.

THE FIX GET TIGHT

Engaging your core throughout the rep is critical. If you brace your core that will help you stay locked into a good body position. I want your body to be as tight as possible and that includes engaging your glutes, your lats and your legs.

THE FLAW POOR ARM POSITION

You don't want your hands to be too far apart or your elbows to flare out to the sides because then you won't get a proper range of motion and you may experience pain in the wrist, elbow and shoulder.

THE FIX GO SHOULDER WIDTH

Place your hands roughly shoulder-width apart and 'screwed' hard into the ground, and keep your forearms vertical as you lower. That will enable your shoulder joints to perform smooth, pain-free reps.

THE FLAW POOR REP EXECUTION

You've probably seen people doing press-ups that look like they are doing an impression of a hen at feeding time. They drop and bounce up and there's no tension on the target muscle.

THE FIX TAKE CONTROL

Take control of your body and movement. Lower under control while maximising full-body tension throughout, with your glutes squeezed, midsection tight and forearms as vertical as possible.

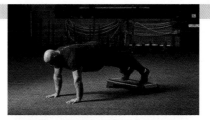

PRESS-UP PROGRESSIONS

DECLINE PRESS-UP

I like to bring variety to press-ups. For some people, regular press-ups will provide more than enough stimulus but others may need more of a challenge so it's always good to have regressions and progressions that you can use. The key difference between the standard press-up and the decline press-up is that the latter works your upper chest and front delts a bit more and is also a bit more of a challenge. I also find that raising your feet increases the core recruitment because it takes more effort to keep your hips up. The height of the elevation is a key consideration. At entry level, you can use a Reebok step box or something similar, and your goal is to use a gym bench. You don't need to go higher than that.

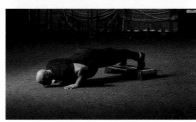

PRESS-UP WITH CHAINS

If I want to overload someone on a press-up movement then the easiest way is to add external resistance. Vests tend to be expensive, particularly if you're buying a range of weights and the adjustable ones can take time to set up. Plates on your back may look cool but they require a partner and it can take too long to set up with multiple plates. I prefer chains because you can place them across your back yourself and if they slip off they're unlikely to cause injury.

The placement of the chains is key. They should be across your upper back as opposed to your lower back. That's the area we want to overload. If you place them lower down then you get increased core activation but you end up challenging the core more than the triceps, chest and shoulders and that's not the purpose of this exercise. You don't need to get too ambitious with the weight. Adding one or two chains is about 10-15kg of extra load and that should be plenty.

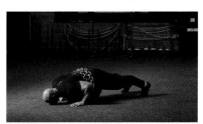

REGRESSION

While bodyweight drills are the goal for horizontal pressing, I regularly supplement these with a high volume of dumbbell bench pressing during the foundation phase. This is particularly the case if an individual is struggling to hit even one solid press-up rep. Dumbbell bench pressing builds your shoulders, triceps and pecs to better facilitate progression on the bodyweight press-up.

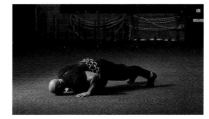

Vertical press

KEY MOVE SINGLE-ARM DUMBBELL PRESS

TARGET
The single-arm press isn't about the load. The key is to be equally strong on both sides and to focus on perfecting technique.

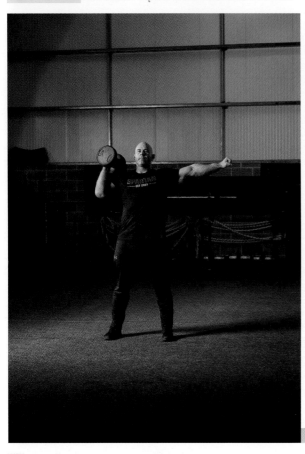

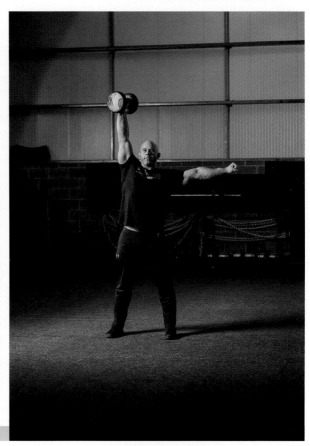

When you come to vertical pressing in the foundation phase, I prefer clients to use a dumbbell and start with a one-arm press. It's easier to press a dumbbell than it is to press a barbell because you don't need the wrist flexibility required to use a 'clean' grip.

I get clients to start with a neutral grip because it's kinder on the shoulder joint. With the unilateral version you get the added bonus of enhanced core and oblique strength because you're required to stabilise the weight overhead, but also on one side only. Promoting unilateral strength can also reduce strength imbalances between limbs.

Clients may not start heavy but that's fine by me. How you move the load throughout the movement is what matters most at this stage. The load lifted is not as important to me as how the load is moved – technique quality is always the priority. Once you've perfected the unilateral version we move to bilateral. That will strengthen the shoulders, triceps and core musculature further and prepare you for the barbell version.

PERFECT FORM

- Stand with your feet just wider than shoulder-width apart. Secure a single dumbbell in one hand using a neutral grip with your elbow tucked tightly in to your body. The back of the dumbbell can rest on your shoulder. Opposite arm outstretched for counterbalance.
- Ensure the outstretched arm is rigid with a tight fist. This will create greater tension through the whole torso.
- Press the dumbbell up smoothly in a straight line. Pause at the top, then lower under control, pulling the weight back onto your shoulder in a tightly packed position.

COACHING MASTERCLASS

THE FLAW INCORRECT GRIP
It's crucial that you use the correct grip to minimise the stress on your shoulder joint.

THE FIX USE A NEUTRAL GRIP
Using a neutral grip, with your palm facing the side of your head at the start, will be kind to your shoulder, elbow and wrist joints. This foundation section involves lots of pressing movements so we need to protect your joint health.

THE FLAW NARROW FEET
If your feet are too narrow then you're not giving yourself a solid base of support.

THE FIX TAKE A WIDER STANCE
Your feet should be slightly wider than shoulder-width apart. The weight you're pressing is on one side of your body, which will try to pull you out of alignment. I want you torso to be as rigid as possible because that helps to provide a solid platform.

THE FLAW THOUGHTLESS FREE HAND
Your free arm isn't lifting a weight but that shouldn't mean it's just flapping around.

THE FIX MAKE IT COUNT
I want to see your free arm extended out to the side and I want it to be as rigid as possible. I also want you to make a fist with your hand to really contract the muscles on that side of your body.

SINGLE-ARM DUMBBELL PRESS PROGRESSION

DUMBBELL PRESS

- Stand with your feet just outside shoulder-width apart and two dumbbells secured at shoulder height. Neutral grip is my preference, though pronated (palms facing forwards) is fine too.
- Brace your entire torso hard, ensuring you don't lean back, and press the dumbbells smoothly above your head.
- When pressing, make sure to engage the lower-body musculature too. Contract your glutes and quads tightly to provide a more stable platform to press from.
- Pause with both arms locked out overhead. The dumbbells can come close but do not let them clash. Exercise caution at all times.
- Lower under control, pulling the dumbbells back onto your shoulder in a tightly packed position.

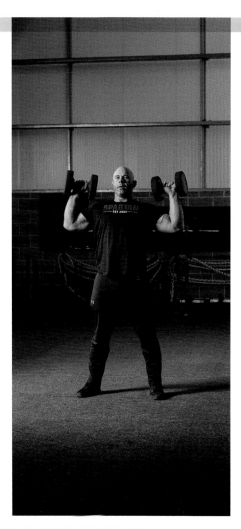
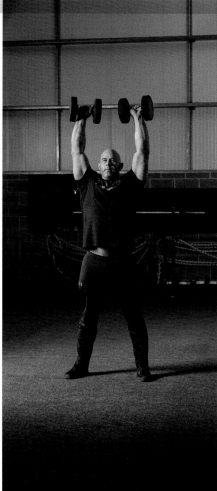

Horizontal pull

KEY MOVE SUSPENDED INVERTED ROW

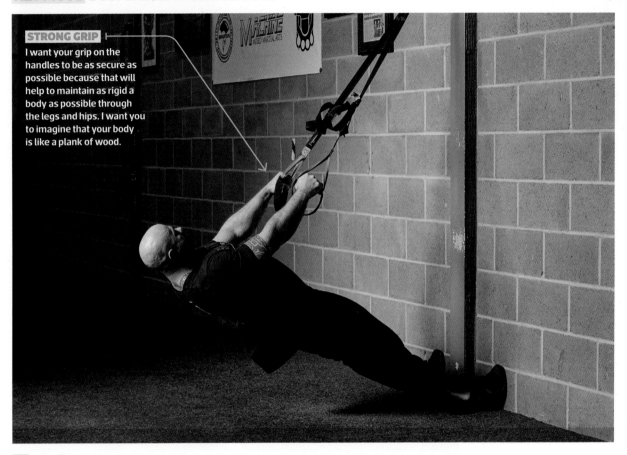

STRONG GRIP
I want your grip on the handles to be as secure as possible because that will help to maintain as rigid a body as possible through the legs and hips. I want you to imagine that your body is like a plank of wood.

You want to develop a balanced physique, so if you are pressing in high volume, then you should be pulling in high volume too, especially in the horizontal pull. Pulling movements are not only the foundation of strong and visually arresting back development but also a great way to reduce the chances of shoulder injuries and impeded performance.

For example, back musculature plays a key role in the barbell bench press. Rear delts act to stabilise the weight during the eccentric phase of the lift, ie as you lower the bar. The same can be said of the lats, which must also be kept under tension during the eccentric phase in order to develop the foundation required to press heavier weights in a stronger and more stable manner.

I like to start clients off with a suitable variation of the bodyweight inverted row, because if you can't control your own body then why would you add external resistance? And if you

don't master your own bodyweight now then it becomes very hard to do so further down the line. For these variations I like to use a suspension training device which is a highly scalable tool that allows you to adjust the amount of bodyweight you're pulling by altering the distance from the wall or anchor point. Another reason I like them is because they force you to maintain tension in your body and keep your core engaged, improving both body awareness and midline stability.

Another benefit is that you don't have your hands in a fixed position – you can rotate your grip as you pull, which is both forgiving on the joints and a tremendous grip strengthener. Grip development is always a bonus. I've never met anyone who suffered because their grip was too strong.

TARGET
10+ reps
When your feet are directly below the anchor point you should be able to do 10 reps.

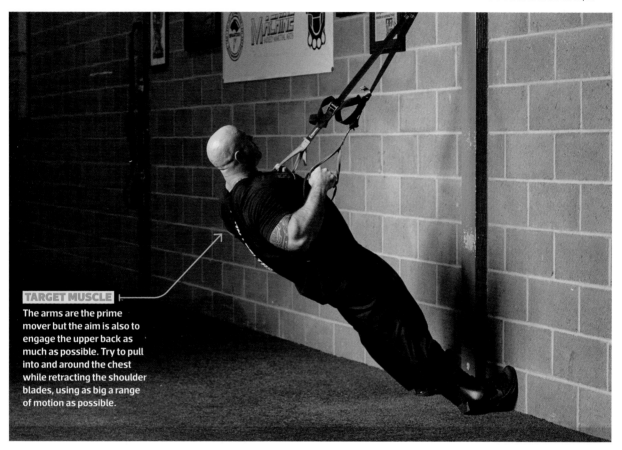

TARGET MUSCLE
The arms are the prime mover but the aim is also to engage the upper back as much as possible. Try to pull into and around the chest while retracting the shoulder blades, using as big a range of motion as possible.

PERFECT FORM

- Hold a ring or suspension training device handle in each hand and position your body in a straight line at a 30-45° angle to the floor with your heels on the floor and your arms straight.
- Engage your abs and glutes, keeping your elbows tucked in to your sides, and pull your body up so your hands just about touch your chest.
- Squeeze your upper back muscles together at the top of the move, then lower under control to the start. Do not let the hips sag at any point.

COACHING MASTERCLASS

THE FLAW SAGGING HIPS
Whether this is done on a bar or using a suspension training device, sagging hips are a sign that your core is not engaged and you lack body awareness.

THE FIX GET YOUR HIPS UP
You want to create as much tension throughout the body as you can so you need to make a conscious decision to become as rigid as possible at all times. That's how you'll maximise the training effect of the move.

THE FLAW NO PAUSE AT THE TOP
You may be going through the full range of motion for the exercise but if you're not pausing at the top of each rep, you're not getting the full benefit of the move.

THE FIX HOLD IT FOR TWO SECONDS
By pausing at the top of each rep and really squeezing your upper back muscles, you're going to increase the training effect. I recommend holding the squeeze for two seconds per rep. It's a great way of learning to control the movement too.

Vertical pull

KEY MOVE PULL-UP

TARGET
5-10 reps
I want you to be able to do this
rep count for multiple sets.

For the vertical pulling movements, I get clients to focus on pull-ups and chin-ups in all their variations, and my preference is to perform them on gymnastic rings or handles that rotate. These promote shoulder and joint relief owing to the increased range of motion and freer movement of the elbows. They also engage the core musculature to a greater degree than standard pull-ups and chin-ups on a bar because you have to stop momentum during the reps. As you may have guessed, anything that promotes core and grip strength during the foundation phase is a positive.

PERFECT FORM

- Hang with straight arms from a bar with hands slightly wider than shoulder-width apart. Palms facing you for chin-ups, palms facing away for pull-ups. Set the bar at a height that means when you hang from it your feet don't touch the floor.
- Brace your core and squeeze your glutes and legs together with toes pointed, if the height of the bar allows. With your abs and glutes engaged and your chest up, retract your shoulder blades, then pull yourself up until your chin clears the bar.
- Keeping your head in a neutral position, pause at the top, then slowly lower, keeping your lats engaged, until your arms are fully straight.

REGRESSION

Most new clients cannot perform a bodyweight pull-up. To help them achieve that goal I supplement their vertical pulling with a great many pull-down variations to develop both back and grip strength.

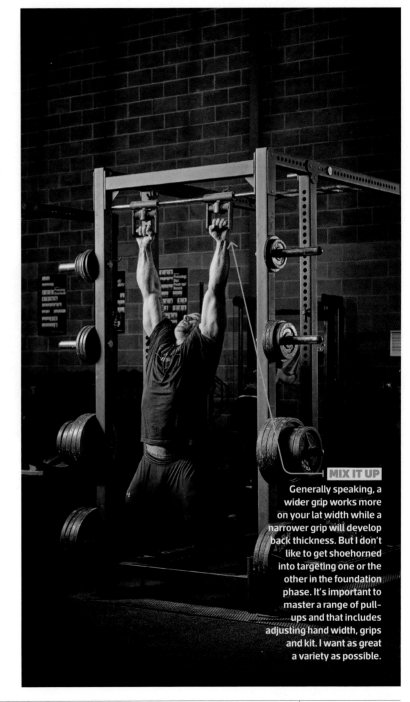

MIX IT UP
Generally speaking, a wider grip works more on your lat width while a narrower grip will develop back thickness. But I don't like to get shoehorned into targeting one or the other in the foundation phase. It's important to master a range of pull-ups and that includes adjusting hand width, grips and kit. I want as great a variety as possible.

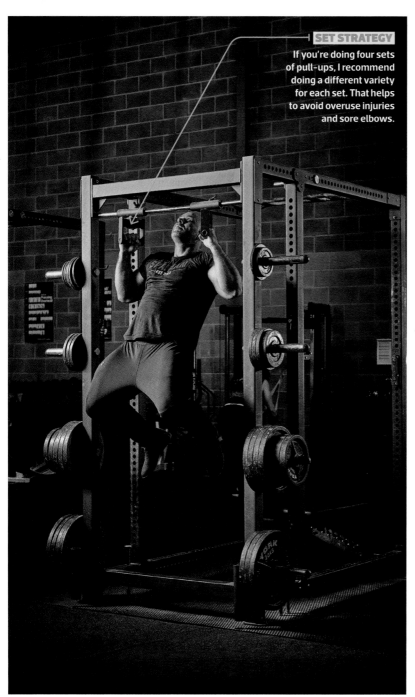

COACHING MASTERCLASS

THE FLAW POOR RANGE OF MOTION
I'm not interested in simply completing reps. I'm focused on how well the movement is performed. With pull-ups it's not a rep unless you go from a dead hang to chin over the bar and head neutral, then lower under control. Anything less is simply compromising progress.

THE FIX QUALITY OVER QUANTITY
I'd take three full reps over six shitty ones any day. Don't get caught up chasing numbers, but focus instead on the quality and range of motion of each rep.

THE FLAW KIPPING PULL-UPS
Kipping pull-ups, where you combine a horizontal swing with a pull, are gymnastic-based movements commonly associated with CrossFit workouts. While a valid exercise if executed correctly, they serve no purpose in a foundation training phase that's focused on learning good mechanics and developing strength in the movement.

THE FIX SEE THE BIGGER PICTURE
Be strict with yourself and focus on traditional pull-ups and chin-ups, which are both challenging and beneficial to upper body development. They can provide a huge return at less risk than kipping pull-ups, while also developing the physical competency to benefit from such progressions.

THE FLAW NOT ENGAGING THE LATS
I see a lot of people doing pull-ups where they're engaging their arms only.

THE FIX INTO YOUR POCKET
Focus on trying to pull your elbows towards your back pockets. If you're struggling to engage the lats, you might need to teach yourself how to engage them in an easier variation of the move, like a seated pull-up variation in a squat rack. The reduced load will help you to isolate the target muscle.

Hip hinge

KEY MOVE DOWEL HIP HINGE

TARGET
The dowel hip hinge is about drilling good technique so there isn't a rep target for this exercise.

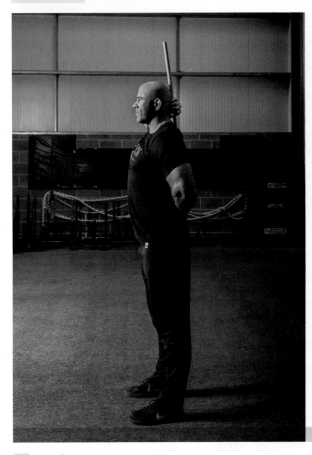

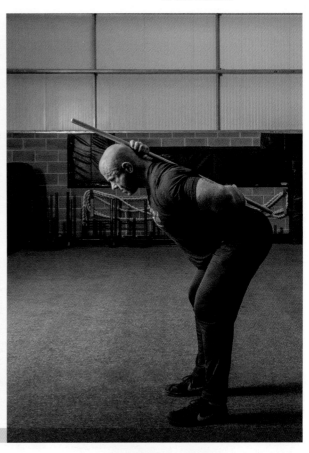

Learning the hip hinge pattern is crucial for anyone before they jump into loaded deadlifts. I like to prepare my clients for the barbell deadlift by getting them to progress through four key variations in the foundation phase. Each individual is different in some way or another and some may skip a progression or two depending on ability. Some may spend longer on a particular movement in order to drill the hip hinge. Regardless, the progressions here are my personal favourites.

I find the dowel hip hinge especially useful as a starting point because it helps the client to stay straight throughout their spine while hinging. The aim is to keep the stick in contact with the back of your head, shoulder blades and tailbone, while sitting your hips back as far as you can.

PERFECT FORM

- Assume a deadlift stance, with feet slightly narrower than shoulder-width apart.
- Hold a dowel behind the back vertically in line with your spine.
- Grip the dowel in the curve of your neck with one hand. With the other, grip the dowel in the curve of your lower back.
- Perform a hinge movement, leading with the hip. Make sure the dowel is constantly in contact with the back of the head, mid back and tailbone.

COACHING MASTERCLASS

THE FLAW LIFTING TOO HEAVY
The deadlift can easily turn into an ego lift so you have to ask yourself: why am I doing it? It's in the foundation section because it's important to drill the hip hinge pattern, not to chase weight. If you go too heavy, you'll limit your ability to hinge effectively.

THE FIX LIGHT AND SMART
When you add load, keep it light and focus on the hinge movement pattern. The hinge is integral for the more advanced training challenges that follow in this book, so ingraining the movement pattern in your muscles is essential if you're to progress to using a barbell and then increasing the load.

THE FLAW NOT ENGAGING THE GLUTES
This is particularly an issue at lock-out. If you're not engaging the glutes you're missing a massively important component of any posterior chain exercise.

THE FIX SQUEEZE YOUR BUTT
The coaching cue I use is to get clients to imagine they're squeezing a lump of coal between their bum cheeks. I want them to squeeze so hard that the coal becomes a diamond. Powerful glute contractions need to be drilled, they don't just happen.

THE FLAW NOT ADJUSTING THE PICK-UP HEIGHT
In the progression move, you don't have to lift the load from the floor to be deadlifting. If your mobility or core motor control is limited, you may find you're unable to deadlift from the floor without losing tension.

THE FIX ELEVATE TO PROGRESS
Start with the kettlebell on a block or low step box. This reduces the range of motion slightly to accommodate your individual issues. As you progress you can work towards pulling from the floor.

DOWEL HIP HINGE PROGRESSION

KETTLEBELL DEADLIFT
The next phase is to work through kettlebell deadlift variations. If you've mastered the dowel hip hinge but don't quite have the flexibility to get all the way to the floor, then you should place the kettlebell on a bumper plate or step box to begin with – that's the method to begin building strength in the movement while improving mobility. Once mobility improves sufficiently, remove the slightly elevated start position and pick up from the floor.

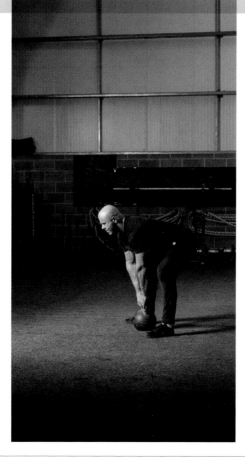
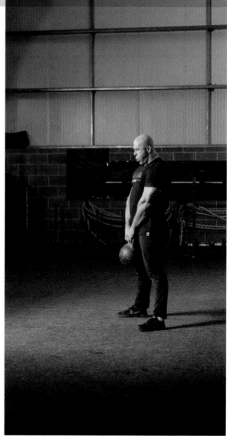

Hip hinge

KEY MOVE KETTLEBELL SWING

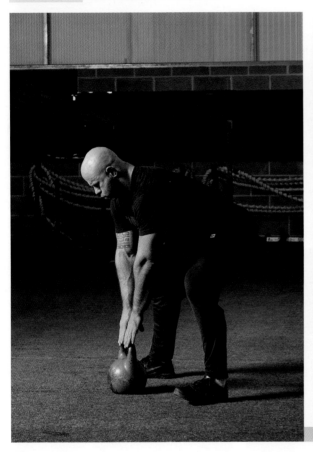 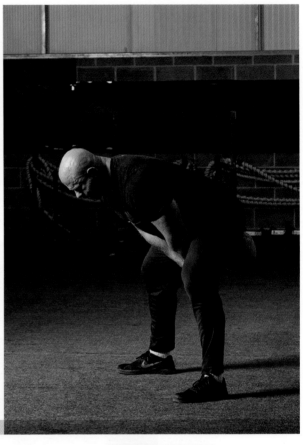

Once you've mastered the kettlebell deadlift the next progression is the kettlebell swing. The swing is an excellent way to add a dynamic and powerful component to your training. Of the two most popular styles of swing, I prefer the Russian style (kettlebell to shoulder height) as opposed to the American (kettlebell high above the head) because it's both safer and more effective.

The Russian swing requires you to start in a loaded position, which is similar to that of the barbell deadlift that we're working towards. To initiate the movement requires a powerful hip extension along with a solid core brace. Ballistic in nature, the movement helps pattern both hip extension and flexion, which are key not only relevant to squatting and pulling but most human movement. The swing does all this while also while encouraging proper breathing and bracing strategies.

PERFECT FORM

- Start in a loaded position, similar to the deadlift on p43.
- Powerfully extend your hips while simultaneously bracing your core to swing the kettlebell up no higher than shoulder height. Your arms should be loose, not rigid and tight.
- As you swing the kettlebell back down into the next rep, make sure your weight stays on your heels, with you chest open and head up. This is a hinge movement, not a squat.

TARGET
Men **15–20 reps with a 24–32kg kettlebell**
Women **15–20 reps with a 20–24kg kettlebell**

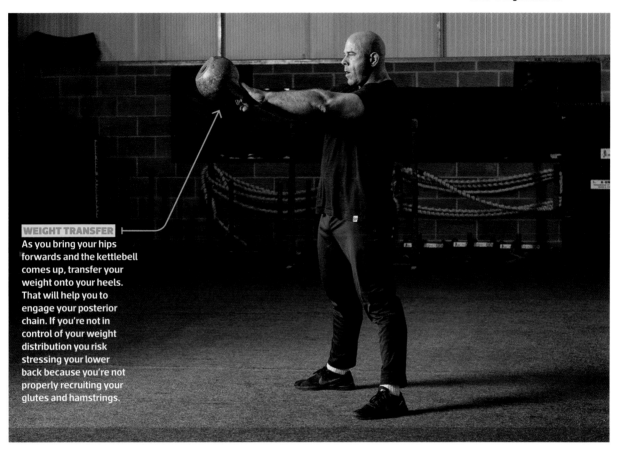

WEIGHT TRANSFER
As you bring your hips forwards and the kettlebell comes up, transfer your weight onto your heels. That will help you to engage your posterior chain. If you're not in control of your weight distribution you risk stressing your lower back because you're not properly recruiting your glutes and hamstrings.

COACHING MASTERCLASS

THE FLAW POOR SET-UP
Many people compromise their ability to swing with optimal form, brace hard and create torque from the outset because they set up wrong. They bend over with a rounded back and lift the weight with their arms only, not their hips.

THE FIX SET-UP RIGHT
The correct set-up sees you brace, and hinge the hamstrings backwards maintaining a neutral spine position.

THE FLAW SQUATTING NOT HINGING
The kettlebell swing is a hinge movement pattern progression. I never want clients falling into the trap of squatting instead.

THE FIX HINGE AND SWING
Ensure you initiate the swing by sitting the hamstrings back and hinging forwards at the hips. When the kettlebell goes between your legs, keep it as close to your glutes as possible. Don't let it drop too low between your knees.

THE FLAW SWINGING TOO HIGH
Swinging the kettlebell overhead as opposed to chest height can see overextension at the top and soft lock-outs with the glutes.

THE FIX GO RUSSIAN
I prefer the Russian-style swing in the foundation phase because you swing it up only to chest level. That way you can focus solely on the hinge pattern and lift more load safely in the process.

Squat

KEY MOVE BODYWEIGHT SQUAT

TARGET

30 reps

There is a rep target for this move – but each rep needs to be technically perfect.

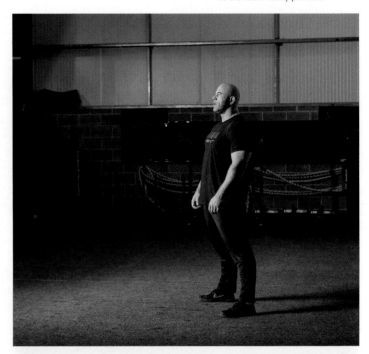

The squat is a multi-joint lower body exercise that is renowned for developing strength, size and power. But in order to reap the rewards of this movement, you must first master the fundamentals.

Just as we did with the previous movement patterns, we start by working with bodyweight only. If you have some level of movement dysfunction at bodyweight only, a useful regression would be using TRX straps because the extra support makes it easier to maintain a rigid torso and balance at the bottom of the movement.

Once you're proficient in the bodyweight version you can progress to the goblet squat (see p48), where the pecs, biceps and upper back come into play because the weight wants to pull you forwards. It's easy to progress the weight so this move should improve strength and hypertrophy.

You'll also notice that throughout this foundation stage the core is being stimulated. In this case you have to brace in the bottom of the squat position. Once you start getting to an appreciable load then your ability to brace in that position may be the make or break of the lift so we're instilling good habits from the start.

PERFECT FORM

- Position your feet just outside shoulder width, toes turned slightly out.
- Brace your core, 'screwing' your feet down as if the floor were butter and you were trying to spread it.
- Keeping your shins as vertical as possible, drive your knees out and pull your hamstrings back to lower into the squat position. When you're stable at the bottom, pause briefly, with hips below the knees and back tight.
- Return to standing, making sure to drive the knees out and keeping your feet screwed into the floor.

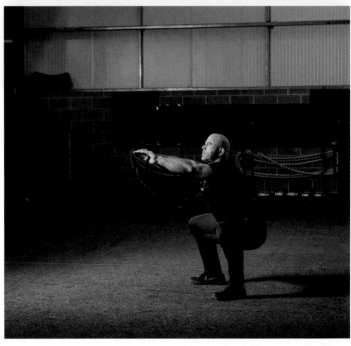

BODYWEIGHT SQUAT REGRESSION

TRX SQUAT

- Grip the suspension strap handles facing towards the anchor point.
- Set up your stance as you would a bodyweight squat, making sure to let your bodyweight pull the straps tight.
- Hold your elbows tight against your torso with forearms at right angles to the upper arm. This ensures your upper back and lats are engaged.
- Squat down in a controlled manner. Your arms can reach forwards slightly as you use the straps to aid with balance. However, ensure to keep the torso both rigid and upright.
- Pause briefly at the bottom, then return to standing. Do not let the straps pull you out of position. It's imperative to keep an upright torso at all times.

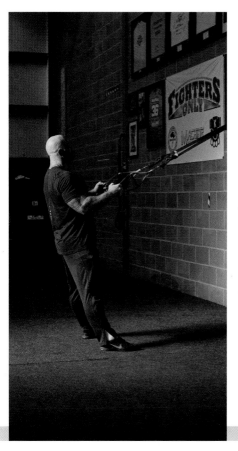
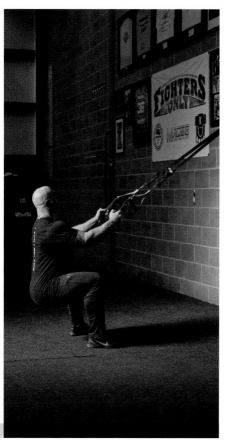

COACHING MASTERCLASS

THE FLAW POOR HEAD POSITION
People who have their head in the wrong position, looking up to the sky, will ultimately end up in an overextended position.

THE FIX THINK NEUTRAL
Simple, but often overlooked: don't throw your head back at the start! Learning what a neutral head and spine means in the foundation stage will only benefit you as you progress to load on all movements.

THE FLAW INCORRECT FOOTWEAR
Your footwear influences your body mechanics and soft, foamy trainers are no good for squatting.

THE FIX GET KITTED OUT
I like a flat shoe, such as the Nike Metcons or Converse trainers. Vibrams are also fine as is going barefoot. The right footwear will help you to stay upright, get into a stable position and avoid unwanted movement.

THE FLAW POOR BREATHING AND BRACING
A solid brace is a skill that is more applicable to a loaded squat than a bodyweight one, but it's a skill that's crucial to master in the foundation stage so it becomes ingrained for future movements and loads.

THE FIX BRACE YOURSELF
Learn to brace correctly from the get-go: glutes squeezed, rib cage pulled down and abdomen tight. Maintain this brace as you lower and pause at the bottom, then exhale as you stand up.

Squat

KEY MOVE GOBLET SQUAT

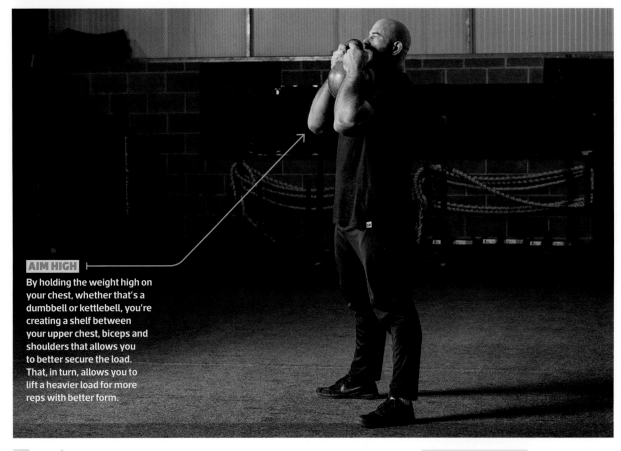

AIM HIGH
By holding the weight high on your chest, whether that's a dumbbell or kettlebell, you're creating a shelf between your upper chest, biceps and shoulders that allows you to better secure the load. That, in turn, allows you to lift a heavier load for more reps with better form.

The goblet squat is invaluable in improving overall squat performance. Yet it is often overlooked, including by myself in my early years of training. If you don't learn to goblet squat proficiently and gain the benefits of its use, then you're going to get caught out when you try to squat with a bar on your back.

Holding the weight in the goblet position against the chest – it can be performed with either a dumbbell or kettlebell – is far easier than it is to have a bar on the back, making it ideal for beginners because they don't have to worry about external rotation of the shoulders. Having the weight at the front

of your body allows you to use the load as a counterbalance to assist in squatting with an upright torso. This in turn forces you to maintain both a rigid upper back and core. Upper back strength and control is integral to squatting with a barbell, while the increased core demands teach you – in much the same way as a front squat will – how to brace and stay balanced and controlled throughout the movement.

I don't advocate chasing huge loads at this stage – we're planning for the future, drilling correct squat mechanics and greasing the groove for future success under the barbell.

PERFECT FORM

- Assuming the same stance as with a bodyweight squat, position the load (I prefer a dumbbell) so it is high on the chest, ideally in contact with both the sternum and the stomach. Grip the load tight with elbows tucked in to your sides.
- Follow the same movements as in the bodyweight version to brace and lower, aiming to have your knees touch your elbows.
- Squeezing the load as hard as possible is a great way to enhance your brace throughout.

TARGET
Men **10-20 reps with a 20-32kg kettlebell**
Women **10-20 reps with a 16-20kg kettlebell**

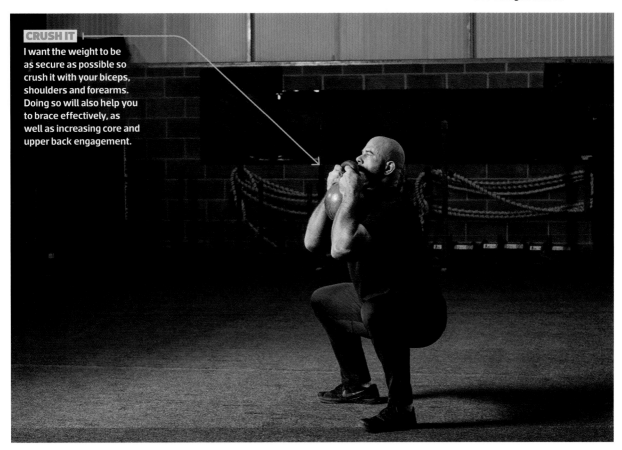

CRUSH IT
I want the weight to be as secure as possible so crush it with your biceps, shoulders and forearms. Doing so will also help you to brace effectively, as well as increasing core and upper back engagement.

COACHING MASTERCLASS

THE FLAW YOU FALL FORWARDS
Squatting down with a load in the goblet position can often see people, even those with good ankle and hip mobility, tip forwards at the bottom. When that happens, the rep is over.

THE FIX SQUEEZE THE WEIGHT
Your upper back and core musculature are stressed hard during a goblet squat. Not only do you require a strong and sustained brace, but you should also squeeze the weight tight and hold it close to your body at all times.

THE FLAW FIXATING ON KETTLEBELLS
Some people think this exercise requires a kettlebell but a dumbbell or med ball will work just as well. It's the position of the load, not the load type, that's important. Apart from anything, if you've got big hands like me, a kettlebell can be hard to hold.

THE FIX BE FLEXIBLE
Dumbbells tend to have smaller weight increase – usually 1-2kg as opposed to 4kg for kettlebells – so it's easier to control the load progression. I also find dumbbells are easier to keep in contact with both the sternum and the stomach.

THE FLAW NO PAUSE IN THE HOLE
You see people squat down and comeback up without pausing. They're not getting the technique wrong but they're missing the benefit of an extended pause at the bottom.

THE FIX HOLD IT IN THE HOLE
I want to get as much as I can out of every exercise and that means being able to make it more challenging without necessarily increasing weight. Performing an isometric hold for 3-5 seconds at the bottom of each rep can be both beneficial and humbling.

Single-leg training

KEY MOVE SPLIT SQUAT

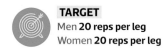

TARGET
Men **20 reps per leg**
Women **20 reps per leg**

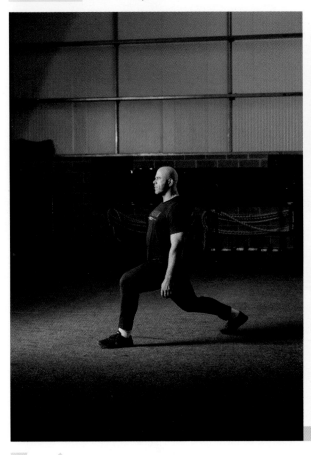

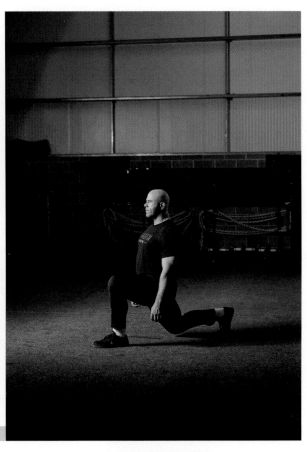

Regardless of goal, everyone benefits from incorporating unilateral training into their routine. It promotes core stability and helps reduce muscular imbalances, and can also help develop and maintain muscle mass, connective tissue and joint integrity.

Performing only bilateral movements such as goblet squats may cause imbalances that result in overuse injuries, movement faults and muscle weakness. Including unilateral training in the foundation phase is a simple way to help negate this risk and give you a more well-rounded base. The three variations of unilateral lower body training that I like to

incorporate into the foundation phase are split squat, lunge and sled pull variations.

I recommend mastering the regular split squat first (both feet on the floor) before progressing to the Bulgarian version, which sees the rear foot placed on a bench, box or step. This progression requires an increased range of motion, places greater demands on balance and stability, and increases both glute engagement and hip/knee stabilisation. It is also easily adapted to emphasise quadriceps (front foot close to the body, knee moves over ankle) or hamstring (vertical shin and lead foot further from body) hypertrophy.

PERFECT FORM

- Stand tall with your chest up and abs engaged and take a step forwards with one foot. This is the start position for the basic version.
- Keeping your chest up, squat down until the knee of your rear leg comes close to or even touches the floor – make sure the knee 'kisses' the floor as opposed to hammering into it.
- Drive up evenly through your feet, ensuring your lead foot remains flat on the floor at all times. Do not tip forwards onto your toes.

COACHING MASTERCLASS

THE FLAW POOR EXECUTION
When performing the reverse lunge (my preferred variation) in particular, I see people step back and then squat down with their weight on the back leg before pushing back up.

THE FIX SOFT KNEES
I cue my clients to initiate the movement by making a 'soft' knee with the front leg before breaking forwards at this knee and simultaneously stepping back with the opposite leg, all while allowing a slight forwards lean of the torso.

THE FLAW INSUFFICIENT TIME UNDER TENSION
Often I see people tearing through lunges of all variations, prioritising speed of rep over quality of rep. The result is they just drop and bounce through a rep as opposed to engaging the leg musculature.

THE FIX DON'T RUSH
Maximise time under tension. For one thing this allows the focus to be more on rep quality than quantity. For another it increases muscle stimulation which, in turn, will lead to greater hypertrophy and strength gains.

THE FLAW GOING TOO HEAVY
There's no lunge one-rep max in the Guinness Book of World Records for good reason – chasing big numbers is both reckless and counterproductive here. You'll increase the risk of injury and are unlikely to perform the movement correctly, so you won't get the full benefits.

THE FIX IGNORE YOUR EGO
Seriously, no-one gives a shit what you can lift here, at least no-one with any sense or appreciable lower body development. Maximise the benefits of this valuable exercise through mastery of technique and application over load.

SPLIT SQUAT PROGRESSION

LUNGE VARIATIONS
I get clients to perform all kinds of lunge variations, including forward, reverse, lateral or Cossack and walking lunges. The lunge follows split squats because of the extra balance and coordination required. I generally find reverse lunges are kinder on the knees but if forward lunges are a problem then we look to identify the reasons why. An effective foundation phase covers all bases and addresses any niggles.

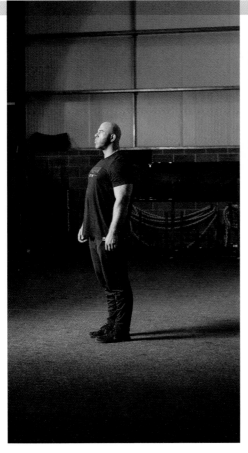
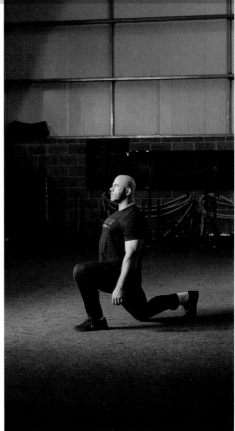

Single-leg training

KEY MOVE PROWLER PUSH AND PULL

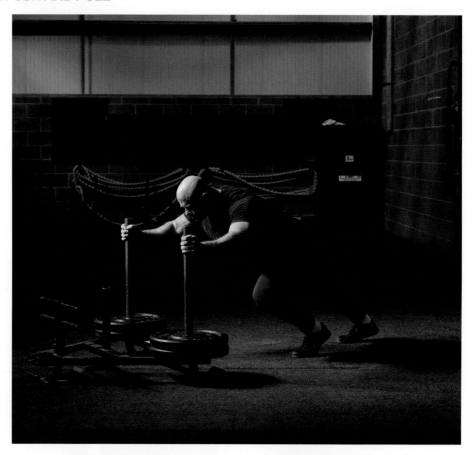

I first had my own sled made around 2004 by Westside Barbell, who weren't too popular with my neighbours when they found they were listening to a metal plate being dragged relentlessly up and down the tarmac! But personally, I've never looked back. Nearly 50% of my facility's floor space is turfed to enable year-round sled training with all clients.

Sled moves are performed in high volume throughout the foundation phase thanks to their accessibility. Nearly everyone can perform them regardless of ability level, background or goal. A sled is a superb tool for developing strength, power, muscle mass, endurance and body composition and most importantly increasing overall general physical preparedness. They get you fit to train in a very short time if used frequently.

They are also a great way to increase the volume of heavy lower body training without increasing injury risk. As with lunges, I get people to perform all variations of pull – forwards, backwards and lateral.

PERFECT FORM PUSH

- Prowler pushes require a track of at least 10m but more is better.
- Gripping the vertical poles, lean into the prowler and move forwards with a powerful leg drive. Ideally your hands will be positioned higher than your hips as you adopt a slight forward lean.
- Strong and determined steps are required at all times.

PERFECT FORM PULL

- Stand at the start of a track – again, at least 10m long – in front of a prowler or sled loaded with weight plates, grasping the straps in a secure grip, thumb over forefinger. Don't wrap the straps around your wrists – I like to stimulate grip strength at every opportunity.
- Start with small steps, pulling either forwards or backwards as required. Avoid any lateral movement as you progress down the track.
- Backward pulls benefit from smaller strides than forward ones. The key is to maintain smooth and assertive momentum down the track.

TARGET
I can't advise a distance or load target because equipment and surfaces vary, so focus on good form with no lateral movement.

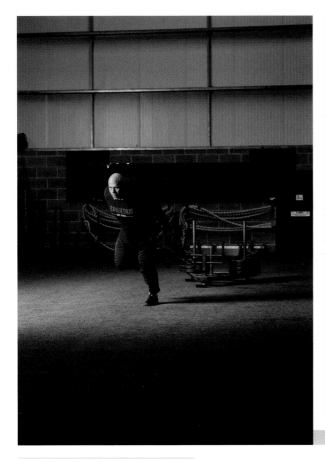

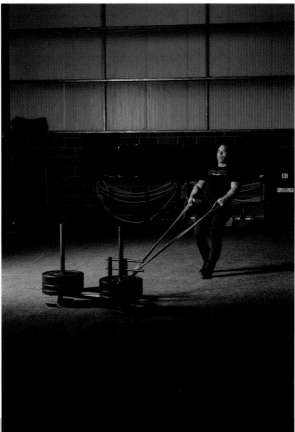

COACHING MASTERCLASS

THE FLAW POOR BODY POSITION
Set up in the wrong position and you'll end up pushing the prowler into the floor, not over it.

THE FIX GET LOW
There are many different prowler designs but whatever the handle you are using, you should attempt to get into an athletic stance with hips lower than your shoulders.

THE FLAW INEFFICIENT STRIDES
If you take too big a step at the start you'll struggle because it's difficult to get the prowler moving well that way. Overstriding results in a less efficient transfer of force from your legs into the ground to propel the prowler forwards.

THE FIX TAKE SMALL STEPS
Start with smaller steps that increase in length as you go. Focus more on the force you put through each leg drive than on stride length.

THE FLAW LACK OF INTENSITY
Performing prowler pushes in a slow and controlled manner can help with recovery and injury rehab, but it's not how you should perform them at all times. I want clients to move as much weight as they can, as aggressively as possible, between point A and point B. That's something I don't see often enough.

THE FIX GO ALL-OUT
The training effect is more profound when you go at maximum intensity, even though you're moving the same load over the same distance. Think sprint as opposed to jog.

Core training

KEY MOVE RKC PLANK

TARGET
Time **60-90 seconds**
I've highlighted a target but it is
more important that you learn to
brace and maintain that brace.

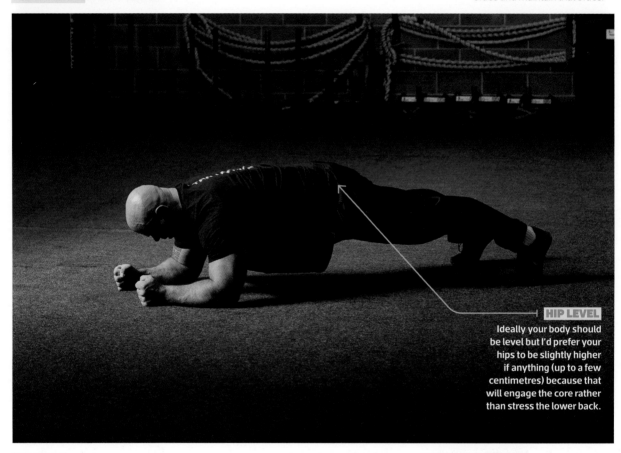

HIP LEVEL
Ideally your body should
be level but I'd prefer your
hips to be slightly higher
if anything (up to a few
centimetres) because that
will engage the core rather
than stress the lower back.

Every move in this foundation stage has an element of core engagement. Why? Because pretty much every client I work with counts their core as a weak link.

When developing foundational strength there are three main types of plank that I like to incorporate into core specific training: the RKC plank, press-up plank and McGill side plank. There are others of course, but I prefer to maximise the return from these bodyweight-only exercises before we add any other.

Sure, it looks basic, but if performed correctly basic certainly does not equate to easy. I encourage clients to push their forearms hard into the floor, squeeze their glutes hard and create tension throughout the full body. I am less interested in time held and more focused on how hard the client squeezes. Tension is key to developing strength endurance in static positions.

PERFECT FORM

- Face down, with elbows and feet shoulder-width apart, support your weight between your toes and your forearms which should be at a 45° angle to the elbows.
- Pull your elbows, shoulder blades and forearms together while maintaining a rigid plank position. At the same time, strive to pull your arms and elbows down and your toes up.
- Hold this position and keep your breathing relaxed.

KEY MOVE
PRESS-UP PLANK

You'll already be working on press-ups in the foundation phase, and incorporating press-up plank holds is a great way to accentuate their training effect and work on weakness. Usually I see people fail in press-ups because they start to drop their hips, and their core usually burns out before their chest, triceps and shoulders do. Using the press-up plank I get clients to keep their hips high to engage the core. We're aiming to be able to hold the position for up to two minutes. After all, if you can't hold a press-up plank for 30 seconds, how many press-ups do you think you're going to be able to do? And remember, I want a good press-up rep to take between four to six seconds.

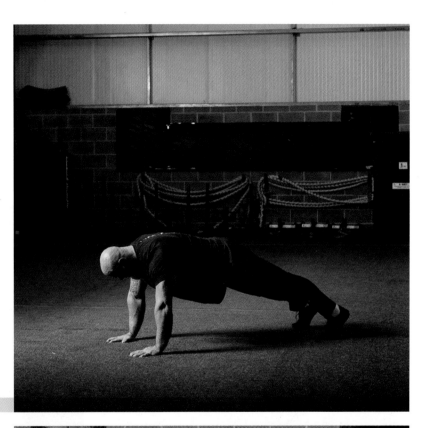

KEY MOVE
McGILL SIDE PLANK

I'd be remiss if my foundational core training ignored the invaluable contributions of Dr Stuart McGill. I've studied the vast riches of his research and practice and I like to incorporate this move, one of his 'Big 3' stabilisation exercises, during this phase. I get clients to keep their legs locked straight and their free hand on their shoulder, as pictured. Staying as tight as possible is crucial, especially in the glutes. Per McGill's recommendation, you should hold these planks for sets of 10-second hard contractions, no longer.

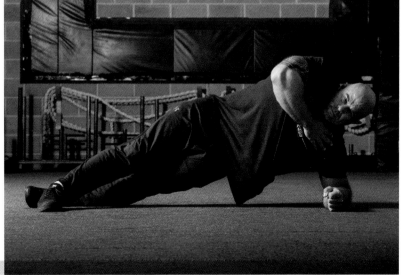

Loaded carry

KEY MOVE FARMER'S WALK

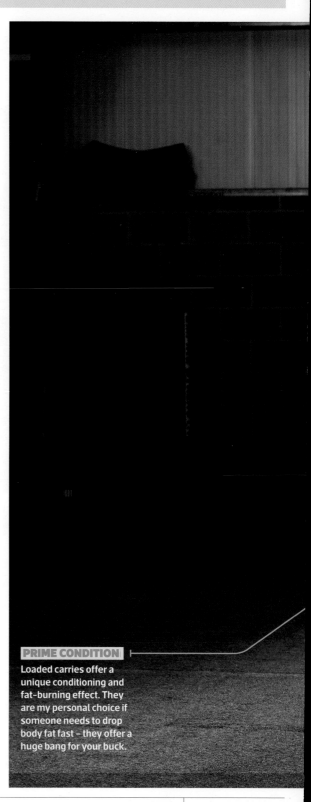

Since day one, loaded carries have been an integral part
of my approach to strength training. Thanks to the likes
of Stuart McGill, Brooks Kubik and Dan John they have
now received appropriate recognition within the strength
community. Why? Because they work, big time.

First, they demand a strong core brace, which ensures the
spine remains in neutral by protecting against both shear and
compressive forces. This is supported by McGill and colleagues'
recent study in the *Journal Of Strength And Conditioning Research*.

Secondly, they encourage muscle growth thanks to extended
muscular tension. A high level of force output from all musculature
is required to complete any appropriately weighted loaded carry. In
particular the upper back, forearms and knee musculature benefit
from this prolonged stimulus. While heavier loads carried for
shorter distances yield excellent results, in the foundation stage I
prefer to focus more so on moderate loads for prolonged periods
of time. These still elicit a hypertrophy effect but allow you to focus
heavily on engaging and maintaining a solid core brace throughout.

In the foundation stage I prefer to focus solely on the
basic farmer's walk, ideally with kettlebells because of their
higher handle and pick up position although dumbbells
work equally well. If the client has difficulty hinging and
picking up from the floor, you can raise the initial height
of the weight by putting it on a step box or similar.

Just remember, lighter loads for longer carries at a slower
pace is where the mileage is at during the foundation phase.
We can get heavier and faster as we progress or move into
specific training for a strongman or strongwoman competition.

- Perform the initial pick-up performed with hands to the side and
  a straight back. Hinge backwards to grasp the handles of the
  weights. If mobility is an issue, then pick up from a low step box.
- Brace your entire core during both pick-up and carry.
  In the foundational phase carries should be performed
  with a rigid torso and strict controlled steps.
- If required to turn (on shorter tracks) make sure
  you do so on the spot and under control.

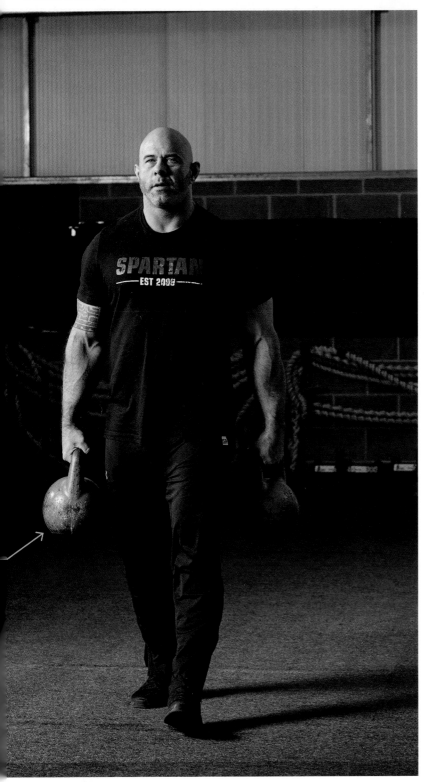

TARGET

I don't use load or distance targets here. It's all about how you pick up, carry and put down the object.

COACHING MASTERCLASS

THE FLAW SOFT GRIP

It may be easier if you hold the load with a soft grip, especially on the forearms, but that negates the point of the exercise. I want the move to be as effective as possible, not as easy as possible.

THE FIX GET A GRIP

If you're using kettlebells, for example, I want you to try to turn that kettlebell handle into dust. Concentrate on gripping the weight as hard as possible – white knuckles at all times – to maximise tension throughout your body.

THE FLAW OVERSTRIDING

Using longer strides will make you less stable and rigid in the torso. You'll also find that you get more lateral movement at the knees and your knees may start to collapse inwards.

THE FIX IDENTIFY THE FIX

Using slower, shorter strides is safer and will allow you to load heavier for longer and get a better training effect.

THE FLAW USING A BELT

I don't want clients to use a weight belt when they are doing loaded carries, especially in the foundation phase of their athletic development. This seriously hampers the core stimulus of the movement.

THE FIX DITCH THE BELT

Using a belt is a skill in itself and the skill we're concerned with developing, at this stage, is your ability to brace and maintain that brace. Adding a belt won't help you do that. I'm not saying that there's never a good time to use a weight belt. This just isn't it. For now your midsection is your belt. Use it.

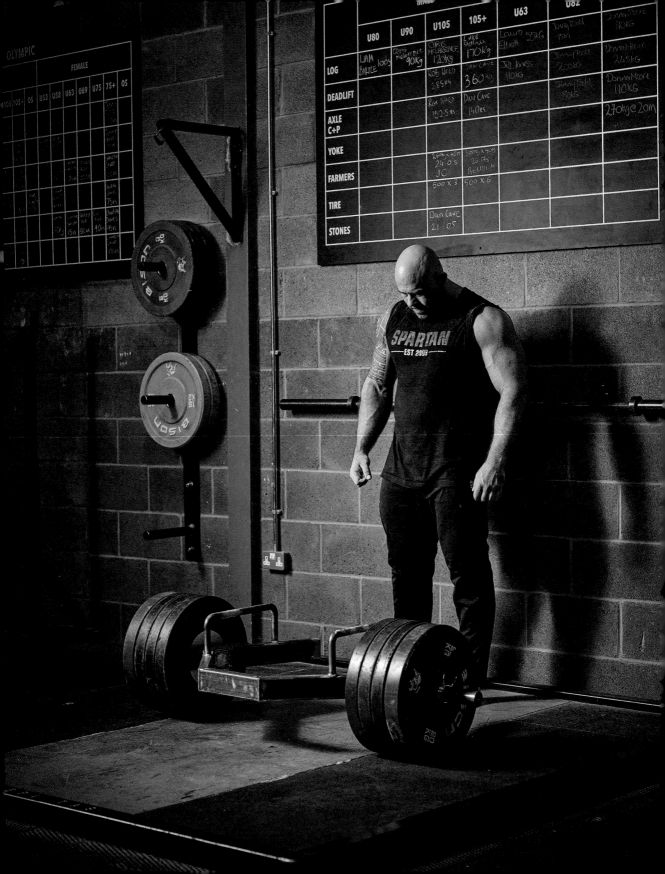

02.

KEY
LIFTS

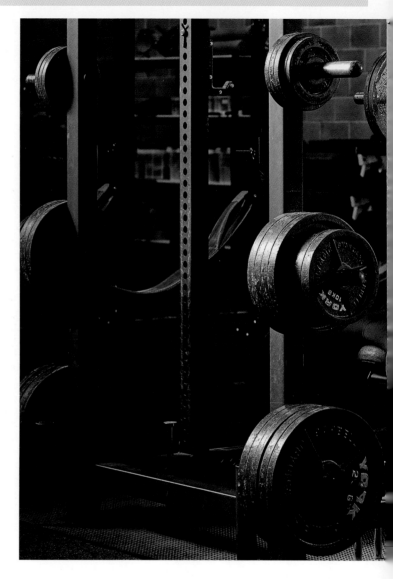

As far as I'm concerned, when strength training you must earn the right to perform certain moves or attempt certain lifts. Only once you've completed the foundation chapter have you earned the right to work on these key barbell lifts.

You'll notice that there are relatively few lifts in this section and there's a good reason for that. This isn't an exhaustive list of useful exercises, nor is it a chance for me to show off with impressive-looking lifts. I don't compete in the YouTube Olympics. This is a list of the exercises that I've found are most effective at developing a solid level of full-body strength.

There is so much mileage in these lifts that you could perform them for years and keep progressing just by adjusting workout variations such as frequency, volume, load and tempo. Of course, at some point, you are going to need to do other moves to iron out weak points or give your muscles a new training stimulus, and those moves are detailed later in the book. But for now, I want you to concentrate on becoming as good as you possibly can be at performing these key lifts.

COMPOUND GAINS

When strength training, everyone is looking to maximise the training effect of a session and use the exercises that give you the biggest bang for your training buck. That's why the moves in this chapter are all compound, multi-joint, multi-muscle exercises. Doing them will increase the efficiency of a workout and it will also promote the release of natural anabolic hormones that are integral to the increase of strength and muscle mass. That makes them the optimal choice for full-body strength and it's why they should be the pillars of your strength training programme.

Once the movements are mastered from a technical point of view, you can start to progressively overload them. This isn't complicated. Want to squat more? Slide another disc onto the barbell and put a clip on. But again, what has to be stressed is that you must first concern yourself with technical mastery before you worry about progressive overload. This is a point

that even the greatest powerlifter of all time, Ed Coan, stresses repeatedly. Technique trumps everything.

That said, you should be able to make good progress because if you have truly done everything you can on the fundamental lifts, lifting the bar won't be a challenge so you will be able to add load pretty quickly. You've already proven that you can get into the positions required so it is quite a shallow learning curve.

COMPLETE MASTER

The reason we focus on mastering the technique for each move is because poor technique will be the flaw that limits your progress. I'm 23 years into strength training and I still work on barbell technique. That's also why I emphasise technical proficiency over targets.

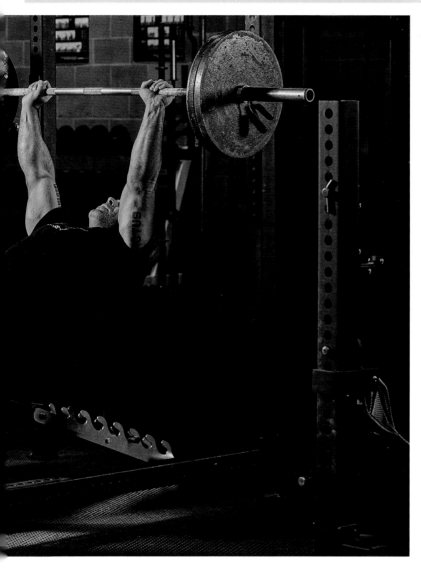

To me, it's about how you lift, not what you lift. In my career, I've never seen someone fail a squat because their legs weren't strong enough. I have, however, seen plenty of people collapse because they lost the ability to brace or because of some other technical shortcoming.

Mastering these lifts isn't just about the movement patterns. It's also about knowing how to brace, how to maintain that brace, and how to maintain a rigid torso throughout the rep. Quite simply, if you don't know how to brace then you'll lift less weight and get injured, but it often gets overlooked as a skill. That's particularly true with men because they get excited and want to rush into lifting heavy. But if bracing before and during a rep isn't second nature then it'll come back to haunt you and remember – no-one gets stronger while they're injured.

If you focus on technique, you'll maximise the amount of weight you can handle on the bar

Takeaway tips

TECHNIQUE COMES FIRST
We covered the importance of technique in the foundation section, and in some senses it becomes even more important when you graduate to the key lifts in this chapter. In theory, you can train these lifts for a lifetime, adding weight slowly and progressively year after year, so it's absolutely vital that you work on your technique. Typically the loads you lift with these moves are greater than with the foundation moves and that makes technique paramount. We can all benefit from improved barbell technique irrespective of experience or training history, myself included.

LEAVE YOUR EGO AT THE DOOR
We live in a world that's heavily influenced by social media. You see cool-looking videos of people lifting ridiculous weights on Instagram and the temptation is to copy them and chase weight at all costs. But if you want to maximise your strength training potential you must approach it as a game for life. It's a marathon, not a sprint, so don't rush to add weight just to satisfy your ego. Lifting consistently and making small steps forwards is what gets results. Ego lifting always ends in injury.

FOCUS ON THE BIG MOVES
Yes, there are many variations of the lifts in this chapter, but I urge you to focus on the ones I've outlined. I want you to spend the majority of your training time on these lifts. It's not like you ever get to a point where a squat or deadlift is no longer useful. If you're smart with your programming then you can keep making progress in these lifts for years and years. And if you're plateauing, you should address that in your programming rather than throwing away an effective exercise. I want you to milk these exercises for all they are worth. I want you to try to exhaust their potential – which is pretty much endless – before you start looking for variations.

Bench press

It's the most universally revered upper body exercise, and with good reason. It has a lot of value as a strength and mass builder for the chest, shoulders and triceps. Even your lats come into play, so if you're looking at training economy it's a very efficient exercise. A compound muscle movement, it will also encourage the release of natural anabolic hormones – that's the case for all of the exercises in this chapter.

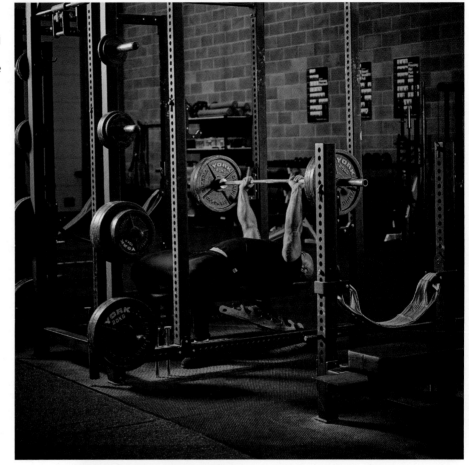

PERFECT FORM

- Set up on a flat bench with your feet planted slightly behind your knees (exact stance can be adjusted based on individual hip mobility and limb length), grasping a barbell with an overhand grip, thumb around the forefinger and hands shoulder-width apart.
- Keeping your chest up and your abs and glutes engaged, drive your feet into the floor and your head and shoulders into the bench to create full-body tension. As you lower the bar towards your chest, make sure it is under control.
- Maintain this tension as you press the bar straight back up over your chest until your arms lock out.

COACHING MASTERCLASS

THE FLAW NOT USING YOUR LEGS
The bench press is a full-body lift so every muscle group should work together. The focus is your upper body but you also need to use your hips and legs. A stable foundation will give you more control over the weight and allow you to press the bar up with more force.

THE FIX SORT YOUR STANCE
Using a wider stance will give you a solid base. People often have their feet too narrow. I'd recommend using a squat stance or wider. Also position your feet so that your heels are behind your knees.

THE FLAW NOT SETTING YOUR SHOULDERS
If you don't set your shoulders properly you won't be pushing off a stable base.

THE FIX RETRACT YOUR SHOULDER BLADES
Use the bar to pull your shoulders back and down. The aim is to use scapular retraction and depression while driving the chest up. This will give you a packed shoulder joint and allow you to drive your upper back into the bench. Driving the bar up too far also ruins a good start position, protracting the shoulders and losing tension at the top.

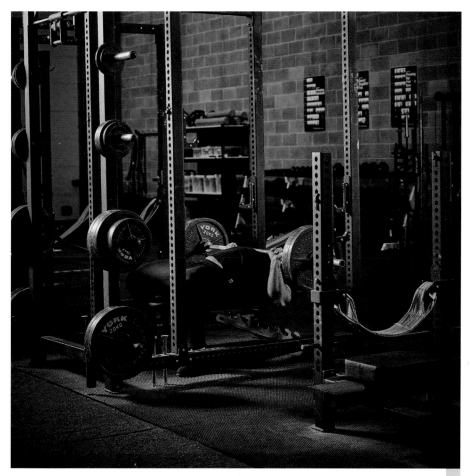

GRIP WIDTH

TOO WIDE

In the example below the forearms are angled outwards, which can put stress on the shoulder joint.

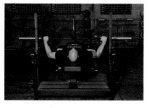

TOO NARROW

In this example the angle at the elbow is too narrow, which emphasises the triceps but limits the amount of weight that can be lifted.

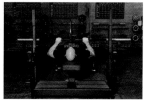

CORRECT GRIP

This grip sees your little finger inside the ring marks on the bar, allowing your forearms to be vertical as you lower the bar and touch it to your chest. Your body type and build will be the ultimate determining factor in exactly how wide you place your hands, but as a general rule this medium-width grip is the sweet spot.

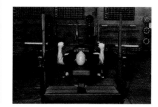

GRIP TECHNIQUE

Poor grip means poor exertion of tension, and poor tension means poor performance. I want you to grip the bar for all you're worth. A tighter grip leads to a tighter body position through a process known as irradiation.

Do not grip the bar with a thumbless grip. It is not secure and the bar can slip from your hands onto your face.

This is the correct 'full grip', with the thumbs wrapped around the bar securing it into place. In this case the bar is too high in the palm, which can bend the wrists back and cause pain.

With a full grip, secure the bar in the base of your palm and close your wrists. In doing so you rotate your hands in before closing them. Make sure you squeeze the bar hard at all times.

Floor press

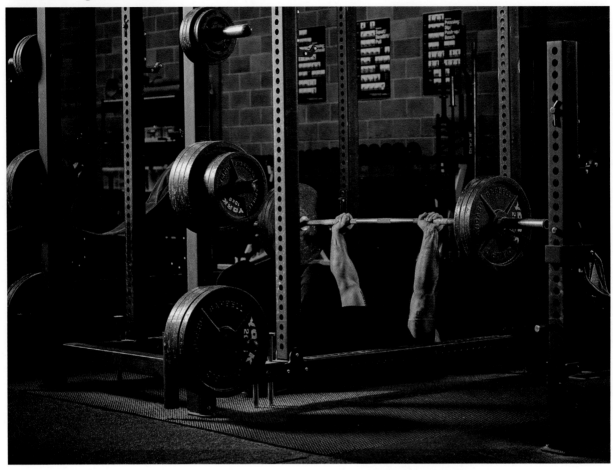

This is an excellent variation and is great for building strength and mass in the triceps, which along with the reduced range of motion will help lock-out power.

Good bench pressing is about pulling the bar down under control and in this move the target of the floor will help you do just that. The static start from the floor will take out the elastic component of the exercise, which will increase your starting strength too. I also find it to be kinder on the shoulder due to the partial range of motion.

It might look like an easier version of the bench press, but I wouldn't recommend it for complete beginners because a floor press means you can, in theory, handle more weight. A beginner may not have the neuromuscular efficiency to do that, so I'd always start with the bench press and then add the floor press. The floor press is going to be an assistance move to the bench, not the other way around.

PERFECT FORM

- Lie with your back flat on the floor with your knees bent and feet flat on the floor, grasping a barbell with an overhand grip, thumb around forefinger and hands shoulder-width apart.
- With your chest up and your abs and glutes engaged, drive your feet into the floor and your upper back into the floor to create full-body tension as you lower the bar under control until your upper arms touch the floor.
- Maintain this tension as you press the bar straight back up over your chest until your arms lock out.

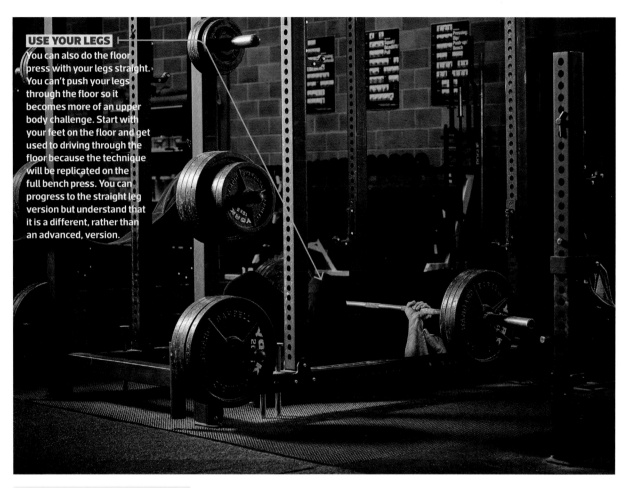

USE YOUR LEGS
You can also do the floor press with your legs straight. You can't push your legs through the floor so it becomes more of an upper body challenge. Start with your feet on the floor and get used to driving through the floor because the technique will be replicated on the full bench press. You can progress to the straight leg version but understand that it is a different, rather than an advanced, version.

COACHING MASTERCLASS

THE FLAW LIFTING WITH YOUR EGO
This is basic. I see too many people, especially young men, try to load the bar with too much weight.

THE FIX FOCUS ON QUALITY
In theory you can lift more because of the reduced range of motion (10-20% more weight than on a standard bench press) but that doesn't mean that you have to. I advocate prioritising quality of lifting at all times to elicit the appropriate training effect. Ego lifting will only end one way.

THE FLAW BOUNCING THE WEIGHT
I don't want to see you dropping the weight or bouncing it off the floor.

THE FIX CONTROL THE ECCENTRIC
I want to see a controlled eccentric and a static start off the floor. Pausing on the floor removes the elastic component of the lift. By not bouncing, you will develop your starting strength off the chest, which is a key reason for doing the floor press in the first place.

THE FLAW LOOSE CORE
Lying on the floor makes you feel stable so it is easy to forget to engage your core, but that will compromise your ability to lift maximal weight.

THE FIX GET TIGHT
You can't engage your legs in a floor press as much as you can in a bench press but you should still keep your torso tight, especially if you perform the move with straight legs. Performing it with straight legs is more of a 'true' lift because you don't have any engagement from the legs. This demands an even greater core brace.

Incline bench press

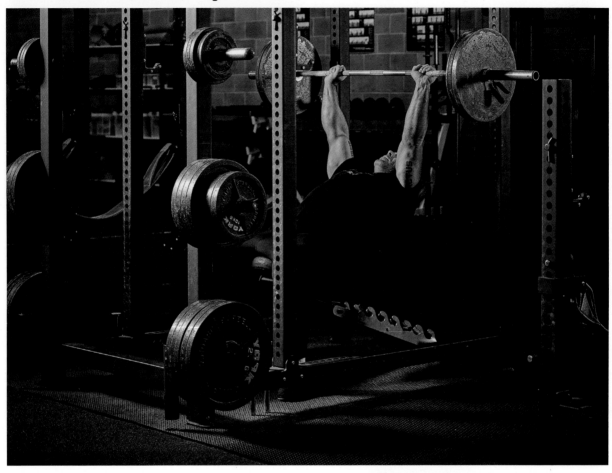

The angle of the bench here means there's more emphasis on the delts and upper pectoral muscles. The benefits are similar to the flat bench press – you simply need to select the right option according to your training aims.

PERFECT FORM

- Set up on a incline bench between a 30-45° angle – I prefer 30°, but this is down to individual preference. Plant your feet slightly behind your knees (exact stance can be adjusted based on individual hip mobility and limb length), grasping a barbell with an overhand grip and hands shoulder-width apart.
- With your chest up and your abs and glutes engaged, drive your feet into the floor and your head and shoulders into the bench to create full-body tension as you lower the bar down towards your chest under control.
- Maintain this tension as you press the bar straight back up over your chest until your arms lock out.

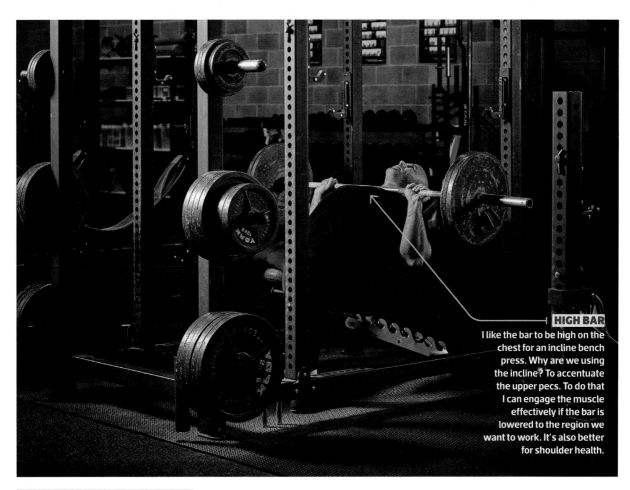

HIGH BAR
I like the bar to be high on the chest for an incline bench press. Why are we using the incline? To accentuate the upper pecs. To do that I can engage the muscle effectively if the bar is lowered to the region we want to work. It's also better for shoulder health.

COACHING MASTERCLASS

THE FLAW POOR BAR PATH
I see a lot of people lowering the bar to bottom of their sternum and not their upper chest or clavicle. If you lower the bar this way, the upper arms angle forwards and the bar wants to fall forwards. You'll feel a strain on your biceps and probably fail at the lift or even get injured.

THE FIX DON'T ROUND YOUR SHOULDERS
Pull the barbell to your chest, making sure to forcibly retract your shoulder blades to keep your chest and shoulders from rounding forwards. Look to actively stretch your upper pectorals as you lower the bar.

THE FLAW FLARING ARMS
I hear a lot of people saying that they get shoulder pain on the incline bench press. This is usually because their elbows are flaring out and putting stress on their shoulder joints. You'll also find that it limits the amount of weight you can lift.

THE FIX TUCK YOUR ELBOWS IN
I want to see your elbows tucked in to your lats at roughly 45° to the body. We perfected this movement pattern in the foundation chapter with the press-up, and we're replicating that here.

THE FLAW DROPPING AND BOUNCING
For some reason, I see more people dropping and bouncing the bar off their chest on an incline bench press than I do with the flat bench press.

THE FIX DON'T BOUNCE
If you need to drop and bounce the weight in order to complete the rep, you're using a load that's too heavy. The fix for this is pretty simple: ditch the ego, drop the weight and perform the reps correctly. Build muscle and strength safely, not recklessly.

Back squat

The squat is sometimes referred to as the king of exercises. That may or may not be true but there's a good reason why it's so popular. It builds mass across your entire lower body as well as in your spinal erectors while increasing full-body strength levels.

It will improve your ability to brace your core and maintain rigidity under load. You will increase your force production potential, which will come into play in the chapter on power training (p108). Remember, the number one way to increase power is to get stronger in key barbell lifts, not just doing lots of box jumps.

I like the fact that you have to be mentally strong to perform a heavy squat or, better yet, a heavy set of 20 reps. Such sets aren't the only way to train, of course, but they certainly guarantee results if you are mentally strong enough to get through them. And if you ask me, the most reliable way to continually improve a client is to work them in areas in which they are out of their comfort zone. Excelling at the lifts you find toughest will make even the most stubborn muscles grow.

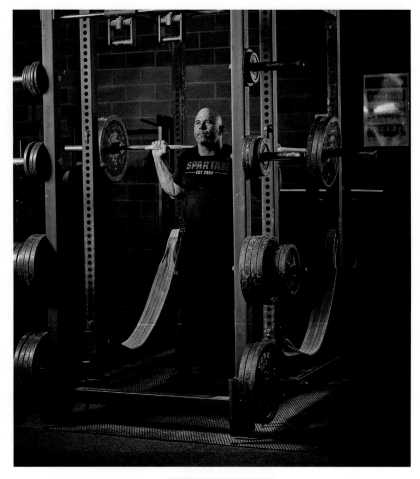

FOOT TRIPOD

When performing lower body barbell movements such as squats and deadlifts, you want the muscles of the foot to work in unison to create stability. The coach Chad Wesley Smith has a great cue for this, which is to think of your foot as a tripod with three key points of contact at any one time during a lift:

1 BIG TOE JOINT
2 LITTLE TOE JOINT
3 HEEL

Equal pressure across these three areas during a squat will provide the most stable platform from which to move heavy weights pain free and effectively.

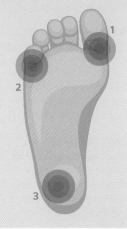

PERFECT FORM

- Set up under a barbell with a vice-like grip and hands roughly shoulder-width apart, securing the barbell on your mid to upper traps. The aim is to create as much tension in your shoulders and upper back as possible. Pull your hands towards your shoulders and drive your elbows down.
- Position your feet under the bar in your squat stance, screwing your feet into the floor, with your toes turned slightly out.
- Keeping your shins as vertical as possible, initiate the squat by driving your knees out and pulling your hamstrings back to lower into the bottom position. Here, you should be stable and pause briefly, hips below the knees, back tight and chest up. Return to standing with a powerful leg drive.

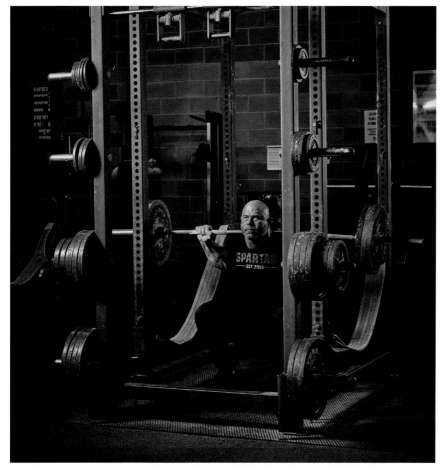

BAR HEIGHT

There are two distinct ways to perform the back squat: high bar or low bar. The key differences relate to bar placement and movement mechanics. Here what's you need to know.

HIGH BAR Positioned on the top of the upper traps, which act to create a shelf for the bar, the bar is more in line with your knees and directly over your mid foot. With the barbell placed directly over the centre of your foot, you must initiate the movement by breaking at the knees first, squatting in a vertical position, knees forward and glutes straight down. This keeps the barbell over the mid foot throughout the entire movement.

LOW BAR Bar placement is about 5-10cm further down the back across the rear delts, behind the centre of your foot. Because of this your knees will not track as far forwards as they do in a high bar squat. With the barbell placed behind the centre of your foot, to stay balanced you must break at the hips first and sit back, leaning your shoulders and chest forwards slightly.

COACHING MASTERCLASS

THE FLAW POOR BREATHING
A lot of people don't know how to breathe when they have a heavy bar on their back. The best result is that you don't lift as much weight as you could. The worst is that you get injured at the bottom of the lift because you're too relaxed when you pause.

THE FIX LEARN TO BRACE
Breathing is an integral part of the brace, which you do to create intra-abdominal pressure. Take a deep breath before you start the rep and brace your abs. Hold your breath as you lower, then exhale as you come up. Take a breath at the top.

THE FLAW USING A BELT TOO SOON
Using a belt properly is a skill in itself. It's not a crutch. If you don't know how to brace without one, you sure as hell won't get it right with a belt. Also, the sooner you use it, the less potential you will get out of it.

THE FIX BE PATIENT
British powerlifter Delroy McQueen advocates using a belt in his warm-up sets when he doesn't need it, rather than waiting until it is too late. But that's his judicious use and experience coming into play. You're not Delroy McQueen. So, for now, lift without a belt.

THE FLAW NOT GRIPPING HARD ENOUGH
You need to grip the bar as tightly as possible to create tension throughout your entire upper body. If you don't have torso tension, you're more likely to fall forwards in the hole.

THE FIX USE YOUR HANDS
I prefer a narrower hand placement, and you should be aiming to bend the bar over your back. Drive your elbows back and down to secure the lats. The tighter you grip the bar, the better your lift will be.

Front squat

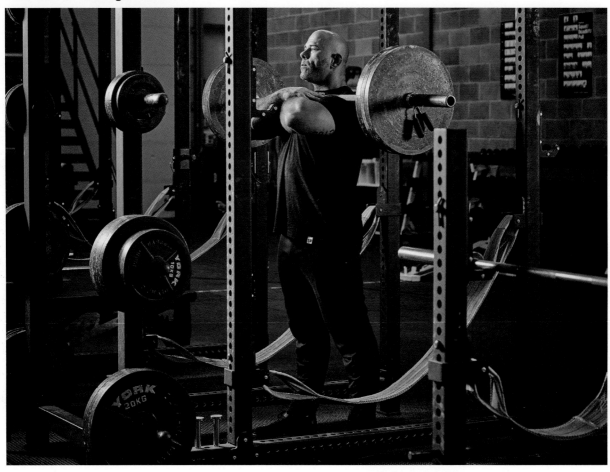

This is my personal favourite squat variation. I find that it's generally easier to get a good range of motion on this movement. You get greater quad recruitment than in the back squat and you have to maintain a vertical torso, so it improves core stability and rigidity, which is usually the weak link in heavy barbell lifts.

Because it's a quad-dominant exercise I find that it facilitates greater mobility of the ankles, knees and hips. It also places a huge demand on your upper back. It's not the best for developing your

hamstrings but that's fine because your programme is likely to include other exercises such as deadlift and pull variations to balance this out.

I prefer to do the move with a clean grip but if that's not possible because of mobility issues, you can take a cross-armed approach. Even though we're not focusing on weightlifting in this book, I feel it is worth persevering and perfecting your clean grip. It has a positive carryover to proper techniques in weightlifting, overhead pressing and structural balance.

PERFECT FORM

- Position the barbell high on the front of your shoulders with palms facing up, elbows up and your upper arms parallel to the floor. If your mobility is limited then variations in grip can be used such as a cross-armed grip, a strap hold or even a safety squat bar.
- Maintain tension by bracing your core, screwing your feet into the floor and driving your knees out laterally.
- Keeping your elbows up, squat down by driving your knees out and pulling the hamstrings back to lower your hips between your feet. Maintain tension at all times. With an upright torso, drive hard out of the bottom position and return to standing.

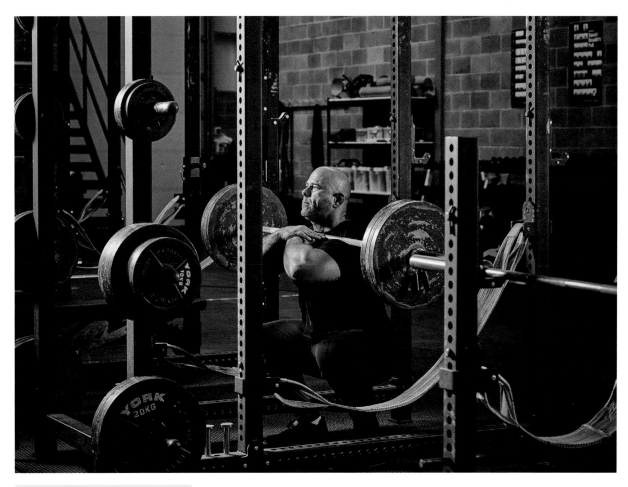

COACHING MASTERCLASS

THE FLAW LOW ELBOWS
If your elbows drop then the weight will fall forwards.

THE FIX THINK 'ELBOWS UP'
Keep your elbows up so your upper arms remain approximately parallel to the floor throughout. The goal here is to keep the torso as upright as possible. A simple 'elbows up' cue can go a long way in ensuring this.

THE FLAW TIPPING FORWARDS
Allowing the body to tip forwards during the lift causes a loss of stability. Not only will your force output drop, but your shoulders, back and knees may suffer in the process.

THE FIX ADJUST THE ANGLES
Elevate your heels. Olympic lifting shoes have an elevated heel. If not using them, simply place small discs (5kg) under the heels. Raised heels allow you to sit back into your hips during the squat, reducing forward lean.

THE FLAW WRIST PAIN
Sometimes the clean grip causes too much wrist pain to ignore.

THE FIX USE VARIATIONS
Sure, mobility drills will help, but unless you are an Olympic lifter you don't have to use this grip and no other. Consider either the cross-body (bodybuilder) grip, strap grip, or even the Frankenstein (hands-free) grip. All are valid alternatives that are kinder on the wrists.

Zercher squat

This is another personal favourite and one of the toughest variations of the squat because of the high demand on your upper back and the compression at the elbows. It offers a unique way to strengthen the squat without the compressive force on your spine. The load of a back or front squat is generally heavier, and the bar position causes more spinal compression.

It can be uncomfortable to hold the bar, so I prefer to use an axle or log. These are kinder on your elbows thanks to their larger circumference and surface area.

Because the bar is in front of your body, there is a tremendous posterior chain and core engagement too. You also tend to get a good range of motion, and this is a good coaching tool for learning to maintain a solid brace for reps.

PERFECT FORM

- Hold the barbell in the crook of your arms with your forearms perpendicular to the ground and your palms turned towards your face, arms flexed. Position your feet just outside shoulder width, with your toes turned slightly out.
- Brace your core and pull the bar in to your torso as you prepare to squat down. When doing so ensure your elbows can be placed inside your knees, which will be driven out laterally.
- Maintain an upright torso, barbell squeezed in to your midsection throughout. Your core musculature will be working overtime if you do this.
- With an upright torso, drive hard out of the bottom position and return to standing, keeping the barbell tight to the body at all times.

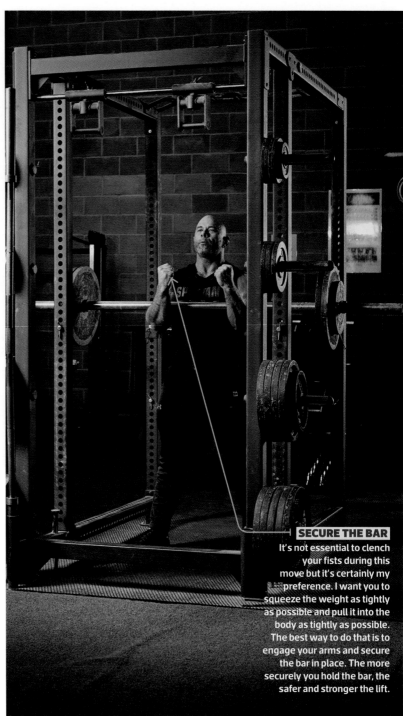

SECURE THE BAR
It's not essential to clench your fists during this move but it's certainly my preference. I want you to squeeze the weight as tightly as possible and pull it into the body as tightly as possible. The best way to do that is to engage your arms and secure the bar in place. The more securely you hold the bar, the safer and stronger the lift.

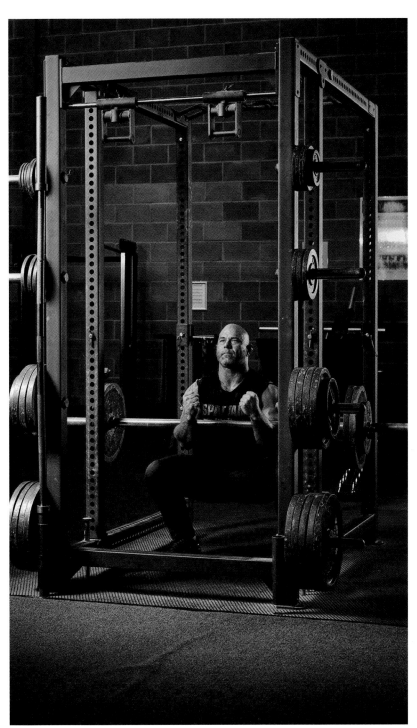

COACHING MASTERCLASS

THE FLAW NOT DOING THEM

Zercher squats get a bad rep in some corners of the strength training community, and as a result, a lot of people avoid them. I personally find them invaluable and include them in clients' programmes frequently.

THE FIX GET LIFTING

The Zercher squat offers a range of unique benefits, including increased core activation, increased range of motion, upper back development and increased biceps and chest strength. It's a great tool and should be used accordingly.

THE FLAW USING A THIN BAR

Using a thin bar to perform Zercher squats will limit the weight you can lift. It has more potential to cause pain and may even put you off doing them altogether.

THE FIX USE A FAT BAR

Using a fat bar will address that issue. Yes, there may be some discomfort but far less than on a straight bar. Better yet, try them using a strongman log if you have access.

THE FLAW BOUNCING OUT THE HOLE

This seems to be done more in the Zercher squat than on other squat variations. They shouldn't look like a shitty good morning. If you bounce out of the hole then you'll lose tension and tip forwards. You'll lose the core recruitment effect, which is why we're doing the move in the first place.

THE FIX STAY IN CONTROL

Lower under extreme control and fight to maintain a rigid and upright torso throughout.

Deadlift

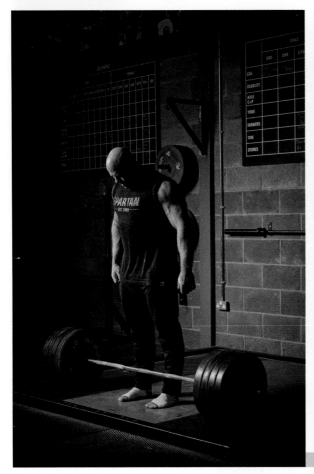

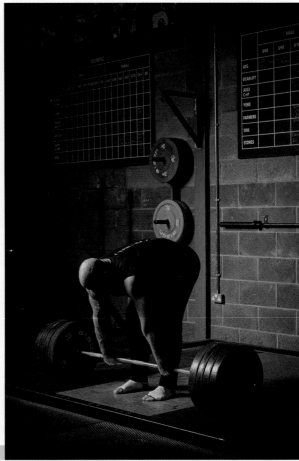

Requiring full-body strength and mental toughness, the deadlift is seen as the ultimate test of strength within strength sports. So does that mean the squat is not the king? Is the deadlift a better exercise?

Well, the squat and deadlift are both valuable in different ways. The squat is a reactive exercise and involves a strength shortening cycle because you rebound out of the hole. With the deadlift you must overcome the load from a dead stop. To do that you've got to activate as many motor units as possible and develop starting strength, all while creating as much tension as possible and maintain a brace.

You want as many muscle groups as possible to contract as hard as possible. Intra-muscular tension is key. That's why I have both the squat and the deadlift in the same programme. They each have immense value and unique qualities.

PERFECT FORM

- Stand over the barbell, shins close to the bar and feet directly beneath your hips. Ideally the bar should be over your mid foot and your feet slightly narrower than squatting stance.
- Perform a hip hinge with a neutral spine until you can grasp the bar. Grip the bar with hands just outside your shins with either an overhand, hook, mixed or strap grip.
- Having secured your grip, brace your core and pull up and back on the bar while driving the knees forwards and out to develop tension in the lats, shoulders, upper back and posterior chain.
- Screw your feet into the floor and leg press the floor away, keeping the barbell as close to your body as possible throughout. Squeeze your glutes from the outset and especially as the bar travels past the knees to lock-out.
- Return the bar to the floor keeping your back flat, head neutral and hamstrings loaded. Reset before commencing the next rep.

EXPERT TIP If you try to rip the bar off the floor you'll force yourself out of a good set-up position. You're likely to lose tension and fall forwards. Your hips shoot up and your lower back rounds. Sure, the bar may come up off the floor faster but your lower back will be in a compromised position.

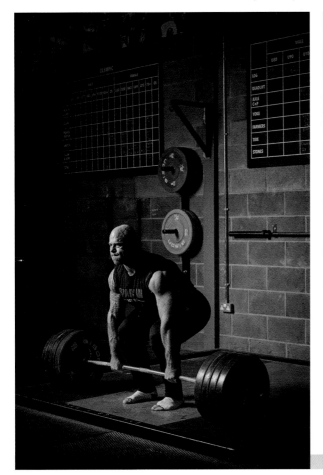
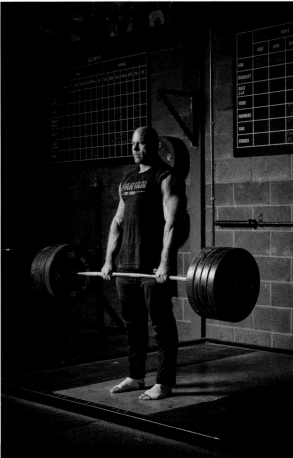

COACHING MASTERCLASS

THE FLAW POOR SET-UP
Start as you mean to go on. A poor set-up for whatever reason (foot, hand or back position) will only lead to either a risky or missed rep.

THE FIX FOCUS ON TECHNIQUE
Technical mastery is your priority at all times. No matter how strong you are, poor technique will always be a limiting factor, especially on the deadlift. Invest the time to master your set-up and the weights will come.

THE FLAW WEAK GRIP
The better your grip, the bigger your deadlift. It's as simple as that.

THE FIX CRUSH THE BAR
You need to crush that bar. I give people the cue 'take the slack out of the bar' just before they pull. If you don't do that you make it two lifts and inefficient. They should be done simultaneously with your core braced and your lats engaged. That way the lift becomes more efficient. A stronger grip means a tighter set-up which means more weight lifted more safely.

THE FLAW GRIP AND RIP
There's a big misconception with the deadlift that it is a 'grip and rip' exercise. But it's not the case that you do it as fast as you can.

THE FIX CONTROL, NOT SPEED
The key is to make your pull aggressive but controlled to ensure that you don't sacrifice your position. I don't care what Larry Wheels does. You can't throw Larry Wheels at me on this. He is a freak and a law unto himself. Neither I nor anyone reading will ever be a Larry Wheels.

Snatch-grip deadlift

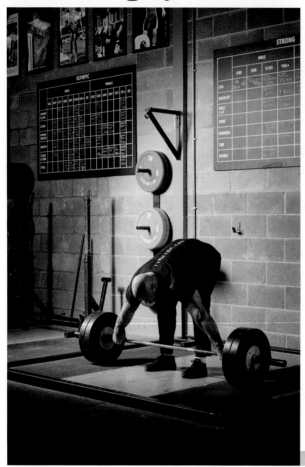
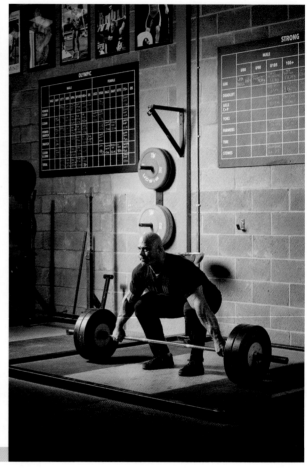

This variation has some influential fans, like the Olympic weightlifting champion Dimitry Klokov and the late, legendary strength coach Charles Poliquin. The wider grip means greater hip flexion and more forward torso angle, which leads to a greater range of motion. It will also give you greater grip strength. Your grip is likely to be the limiting factor in this move so I sometimes use straps. But the stronger your grip, the bigger your deadlift, so I'll also do it strapless overhand or with a hook grip to develop grip strength.

PERFECT FORM

- Stand over the barbell, shins close to the bar and feet directly beneath your hips. Ideally the bar should be over your mid foot and feet slightly narrower than squatting stance, toes turned slightly outwards.
- Perform a hip hinge with a neutral spine until you can grasp the bar (more advanced individuals may do this simultaneously). Assume a snatch-grip-width hand position, using a double overhand grip (hook/strap grip is optional).
- Having secured your grip, brace your core and pull up and back on the bar

while driving your knees forwards and out. Your chest should be pulled upwards, hips slightly above knee level and shoulders slightly above hip level.
- Screw your feet into the floor and pull upwards on the barbell with your back, traps and arms, while simultaneously leg pressing the floor away.
- Your chest must remain high and the bar close to the body as you stand upright. When returning to the floor, ensure tension is not lost at the back and hips.
- Reset perfectly before commencing a second rep.

GRIP OPTIONS The hook grip gives you the potential to lift more weight but it requires technique and pain tolerance. You should be able to lift more in a snatch-grip deadlift than you can snatch, but that means even greater potential for pain. So use it if it allows you to do more reps or lift a heavier weight, although the double overhand grip should be your go-to for strength training because it will develop pure grip strength. Ultimately, I care more about your lifting technique than which grip you use.

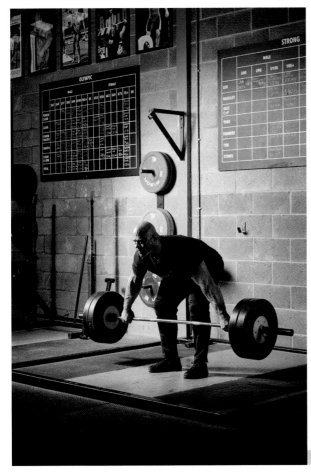
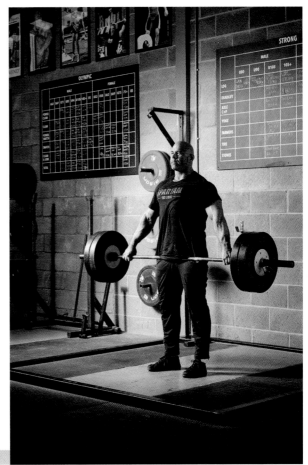

COACHING MASTERCLASS

THE FLAW EGO LIFTING
This is something that I see all the time: people loading the bar so it is too heavy. They miss the lift and get pissed off so they don't even bother doing it at all.

THE FIX BE SMART
You can't lift as much as you can in the conventional deadlift so you need to accept that in advance and embrace the lift for the benefits it can provide.

THE FLAW POOR USE OF STRAPS
Don't use straps too soon. Equally, some people don't use them when they should use them.

THE FIX USE STRAPS JUDICIOUSLY
When your hands are wider your grip will be weaker but it will bring your grip strength up, so why would you immediately use straps and lose that training effect? At some point, however, you'll realise your posterior chain can lift 200kg but your grip can only manage 160kg. If that's the case you'll be lifting sub-maximal so when your grip goes it makes sense to use straps.

THE FLAW LIFTING LIKE A DEADLIFT
This is not simply a conventional deadlift with a wider hand grip. Adjust your technique accordingly with chest pulled upwards, hips slightly above knee level and shoulders slightly above hip level.

THE FIX ADJUST YOUR SET-UP
To get into position with a wider grip, turn your toes out a bit more – about 10-20° to enable your torso to get into a better position and encourage you to keep your lower back nice and rigid.

Trap bar deadlift

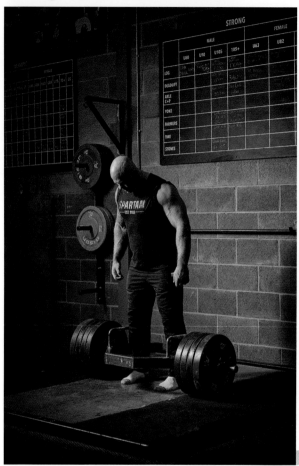
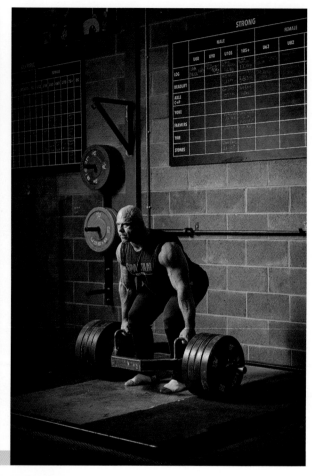

The trap bar is a good tool to transition from the foundation exercises to the conventional deadlift. The neutral grip and central weight distribution help people get into an optimal starting position with relative ease while also being kinder on the lower back. New lifters can develop basic strength and muscle mass with the trap bar as they learn the proper control and rigidity required to deadlift conventionally.

It is also important to note that the only individuals who have to conventionally deadlift are powerlifters and strongmen or women. Their sport involves this specific movement. With all other clients I recommend identifying the right hinge movement for them and their goals on an individual basis.

PERFECT FORM

- Stand inside the trap bar, feet directly beneath your hips. Ideally the ends of the bar should be in line with your mid foot and feet slightly narrower than squatting stance, toes turned slightly outwards.
- Perform a hip hinge with a neutral spine until you can grasp the handles either side of your torso. Your grip should be in the middle of the handles and vice-like.
- Having secured your grip, brace your core and pull up and back on the bar while driving your knees forwards and out. Your chest should be pulled upwards, hips slightly lower than a conventional deadlift and shins angled slightly forwards.
- Screw your feet into the floor and pull upwards on the barbell with a flat back and long arms. Leg press the floor away and keep your chest high to stand upright and locked out.
- To return to the floor hinge your hips back and bend slightly at the knee.
- Reset perfectly before commencing your next rep.

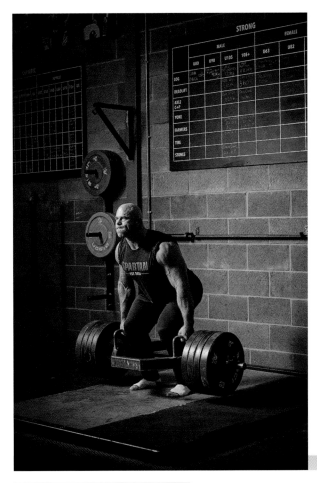

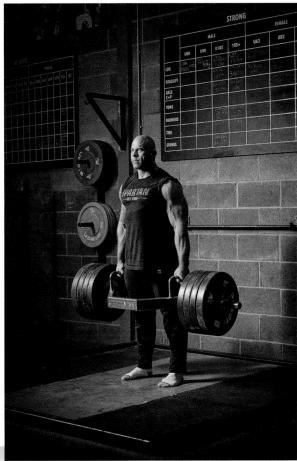

COACHING MASTERCLASS

THE FLAW ASSUMING IT IS A HINGE-BASED MOVEMENT

The trap bar deadlift is like a hybrid of a deadlift and a squat but it is also different from both, so you can't approach it like either of those lifts. Yes, you can get into position with a hinge but you won't lift as much weight or get as many benefits.

THE FIX USE YOUR QUADS

To lift correctly, pull up and back on the bar while driving your knees forwards and out. Your chest should be pulled upwards, hips slightly lower than a conventional deadlift and shins angled slightly forwards.

THE FLAW TREATING IT AS JUST AN ASSISTANCE MOVE

The trap bar does not seem to get the same respect as a conventional deadlift. But if you trap deadlift 300kg are you not damn strong? If you're not a powerlifter then you don't have to focus on the conventional deadlift and relegate other variations to being an afterthought.

THE FIX TREAT IT WITH RESPECT

The training effect and strength gains of a trap bar deadlift are as impressive as a conventional deadlift, yet it is easier to learn and comes with less risk of injury.

THE FLAW POOR HANDLE HEIGHT

Trap bars aren't made to competition standard so they aren't a uniform piece of equipment. The grip width and height can vary between bars. Handles that are too low can be an issue.

THE FIX USE BLOCKS

If the handles are too low so that you can't reach them and maintain an optimal back position, then look to raise the bar on blocks to a height that suits. Better yet, use a trap bar that has handles elevated above the frame, as I do. Don't be afraid to adjust the pick-up height.

Romanian deadlift

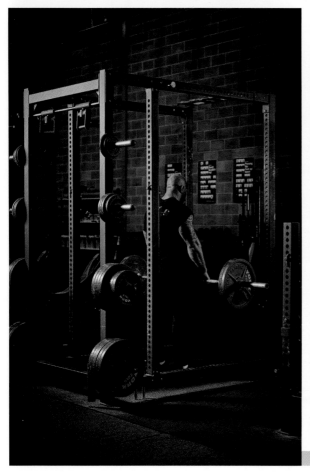
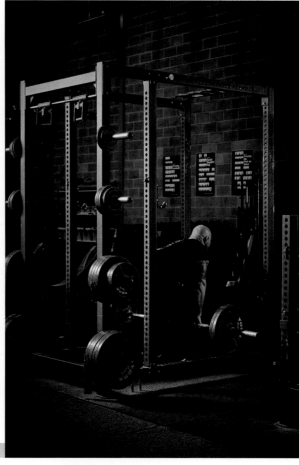

The Romanian deadlift or RDL has been primed heavily during the foundation phase and is one of the best accessory moves you can do for the entire posterior chain (hamstrings, glutes and back). It teaches an effective hip hinge that can be loaded with more weight as your technical proficiency develops. However, I usually play around with tempo, pauses and even adding bands to engage the glutes more as opposed to fixating on getting more weight on the bar.

PERFECT FORM

- Set up either by conventionally deadlifting to a standing position or taking the barbell from a rack.
- Once you're upright and locked out, drive your hips back and load the hip hinge movement pattern, engaging the posterior chain.
- Keep a flat back throughout. Tension should be especially high in the hamstrings and your chest should more towards parallel to the floor, with the bar pulled close to the legs at all times.
- Return upright by contracting your glutes and hamstrings hard, engaging your lats to keep the bar tight to your legs.

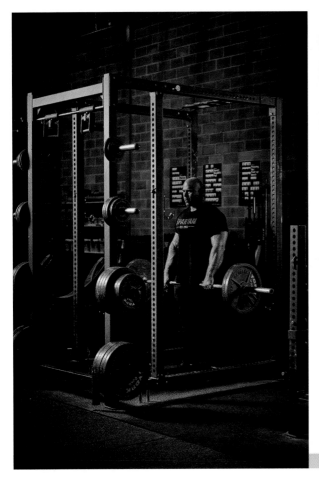

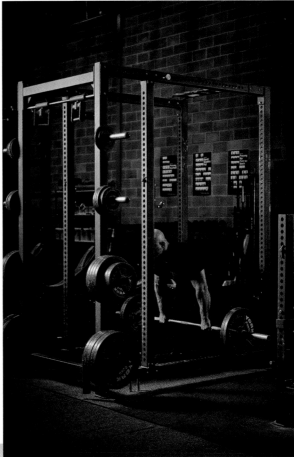

COACHING MASTERCLASS

THE FLAW ONLY USING BARBELLS
We're using a Romanian deadlift to drill
the hip hinge movement pattern, to
improve proprioception and to engage the
hamstrings, but there are more ways to do
this than the old double overhand grip on a
barbell.

THE FIX GET CREATIVE WITH KIT
You can use kettlebells, dumbbells or a trap
bar, which will allow you to take a neutral
grip at the side of the body. They are all
valid options. Choose the method that
works best for you.

THE FLAW SQUATTING, NOT HINGING
Avoid squatting while doing the move.
You might find that you can lift more
weight but you'll be missing out on
the main benefits of the exercise.

THE FIX RECRUIT THE GLUTES AND HAMS
The Romanian deadlift should be a pure
hip hinge movement where you use a
slow eccentric hinge to overload the
hamstrings and then recruit the glutes
in the concentric portion of the lift.

THE FLAW GOING TOO LOW
If you go too low you'll tend to round your
back, taking tension off the hamstrings
and putting it on to the lower back.

**THE FIX CONTROL THE
RANGE OF MOTION**
Go as low as you can to maximise
hamstring tension while
maintaining a flat back.

Military press

Overhead pressing is an often overlooked movement pattern and it happens to be my favourite way to develop upper body pressing strength. I speak from personal experience here. My bench press went from 180kg to 220kg during a training cycle that focused on military pressing with bench press as assistance. During the same period, my military press went from 100kg to 155kg. If you improve your military press, then your bench press will go up – but that's not the case in reverse in my experience.

Because it's performed standing the military press requires a greater core component than the seated overhead press, which to me significantly increases the value of the exercise. If you're pressing overhead, then your spinal erectors need both strength and endurance. Your delts, traps and triceps are all working too.

Despite its benefits I find it a notoriously tricky lift to improve quickly and consistently. You have to fight for every extra rep and every extra kilo increase. That's frustrating for some people, but I love lifts that require mental fortitude. In my opinion, strength training is a game for life and improvements should be measured in years. It's a long game and that's the way you have to look at it if you want to get genuinely strong. That's why I am more impressed when I see a great overhead press than a great bench press.

PERFECT FORM

- Take the barbell out of the rack as if setting up for a front squat, braced and tight before you even lift the bar.
- With feet shoulder-width apart (or slightly wider), secure the bar on your chest, shoulders and palms. Pull the shoulders back, brace your core and squeeze your glutes hard.
- Press the bar directly overhead. Think of moving your head around the bar, not the bar around your head.
- Once locked out, push your head through your arms into a neutral position. Do not lean back or force your head too far forwards.
- Lower the bar under control, keeping your elbows tight, shoulders back and glutes squeezed hard.

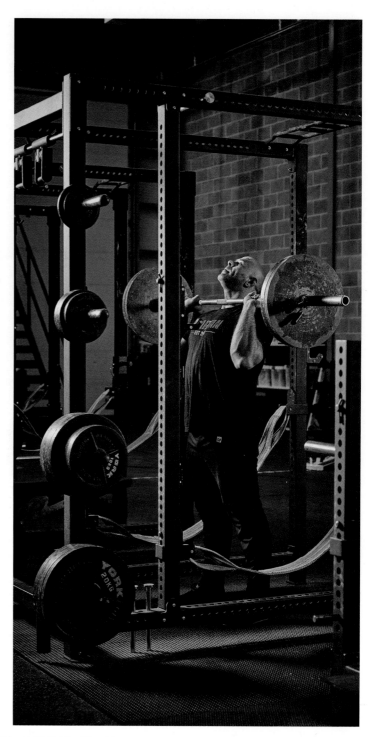

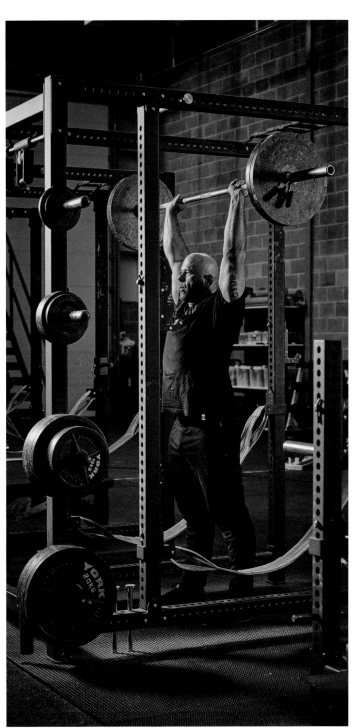

COACHING MASTERCLASS

THE FLAW FEET TOO NARROW
When your feet are too narrow you have a poor base of support. This is even more pronounced than in the bench press because your feet are your only contact point for stability in the overhead press.

THE FIX USE A SOLID STANCE
Your feet should be shoulder width or wider to provide a secure base. I like to think about trying to create a strong structure, like a pyramid, where the base is wider than the top.

THE FLAW POOR SHOULDER MOBILITY
If it looks like you're doing a standing incline bench press, you're doing it wrong. It's also a sign that your shoulder mobility requires addressing.

THE FIX WORK ON STABILITY
You need to make sure that you have healthy, mobile shoulders before you attempt the overhead press. I've known five-plate-a-side bench press guys who can't raise their own hands overhead. Their poor military press strength has nothing to do with a deficit of triceps strength – it's a mobility issue.

THE FLAW NOT PAUSING OVERHEAD
I don't want to see you press the bar straight up and immediately drop out of position. If you do that you're missing out on the potential benefits of a pause at the top of each rep.

THE FIX DON'T RUSH THE LIFT
When you're locked out overhead you have to grip the bar tighter and that places more emphasis on the traps, triceps and shoulders. It increases time under tension and you get greater muscular gains. You could even try to hold the lock-out on the last rep of a set for five seconds. I like to milk every exercise for its full potential and this is one way to do that.

Push press

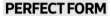

The military press is a key lift, and it's the movement pattern that you ingrain in the foundation phase by focusing on dumbbell press variations, but the push press is also valuable. It's primarily used to develop the delts and triceps, but you get bonus lower body development too through the explosive leg drive.

It also gives you a way of overloading the upper body on the eccentric (lowering) phase of the lift, where you have to control the bar back to the start. Leg drive aids the concentric (pressing) portion of the lift, but the upper body has all the work to do when lowering.

My advice would be to master the military press first because you need to ensure that you can stabilise the load overhead and return it under control. The way I see it, you have to earn the right to use the push press.

PERFECT FORM

- Set up exactly as you would on the military press, keeping your elbows high to maintain a stable position.
- Maintain an upright torso, driving your knees out laterally and dipping your hips. Ensure your feet are screwed into the ground throughout.
- Explosively press the weight above your head by extending your knees and hips, keeping your head out of the bar's path. Keep your elbows in and shoulders back.
- Once you're locked out, push your head through your arms into a neutral position. Do not lean back or force your head too far forwards.
- Lower the bar under control, keeping your elbows tight, shoulders back and glutes squeezed hard.

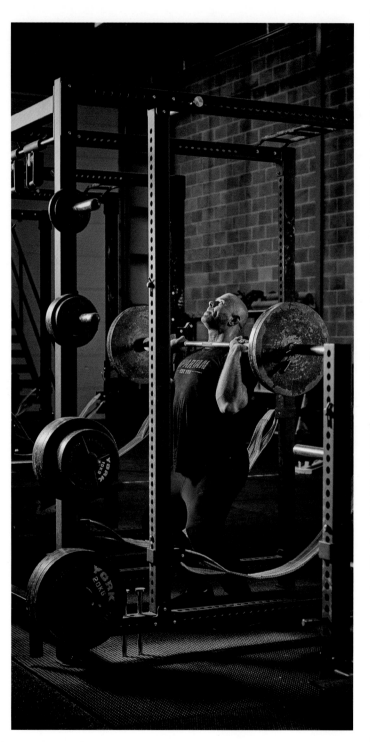

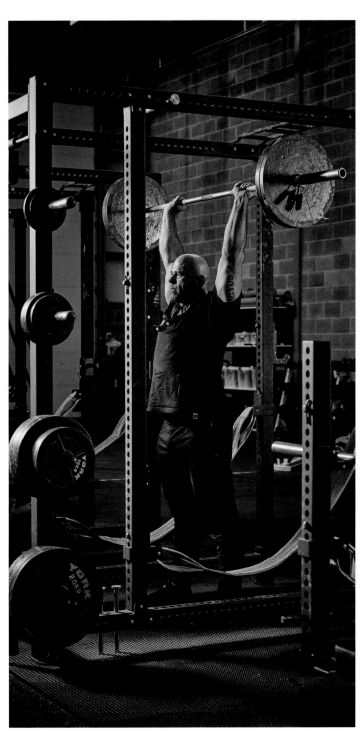

COACHING MASTERCLASS

THE FLAW USING IT TOO SOON
A while ago I had a 180kg push press and an 80kg strict press because there was a flaw in my strength. My legs were strong enough but my shoulders and triceps weren't. So now I advise people not to use the push press until they have perfected the technique on the strict press and begun to exploit their strength potential.

THE FIX EARN THE RIGHT TO PUSH
When you perform a push press, the leg drive 'cheats' the move and the real benefit comes from the lowering portion of the lift. If you go to the push press too soon then you won't get that benefit. Also, in my experience, if your strict press improves you generally see an increase in your whole-body strength and musculature.

THE FLAW DOUBLE DIPPING UNDER THE BAR
If you dip under the bar after you press you can lift more weight. It's great for showing off but it is not a push press and doesn't stimulate the delts and traps to the same degree as a proper push press.

THE FIX BE STRICT WITH FORM
Dip and then drive the bar up using leg and shoulder strength in conjunction. Don't dip twice and reduce the demands on the shoulders.

THE FLAW DIPPING TOO LOW
A push press is not a thruster. You're not performing a squat to press. You only need to dip slightly to maximise your leg drive.

THE FIX USE A QUARTER SQUAT
If you dip too low you'll lose tension in your upper back so the drive from the legs becomes inefficient. If you dip just low enough then more of your leg drive goes into pressing the weight overhead rather than wasting it getting back to where you started.

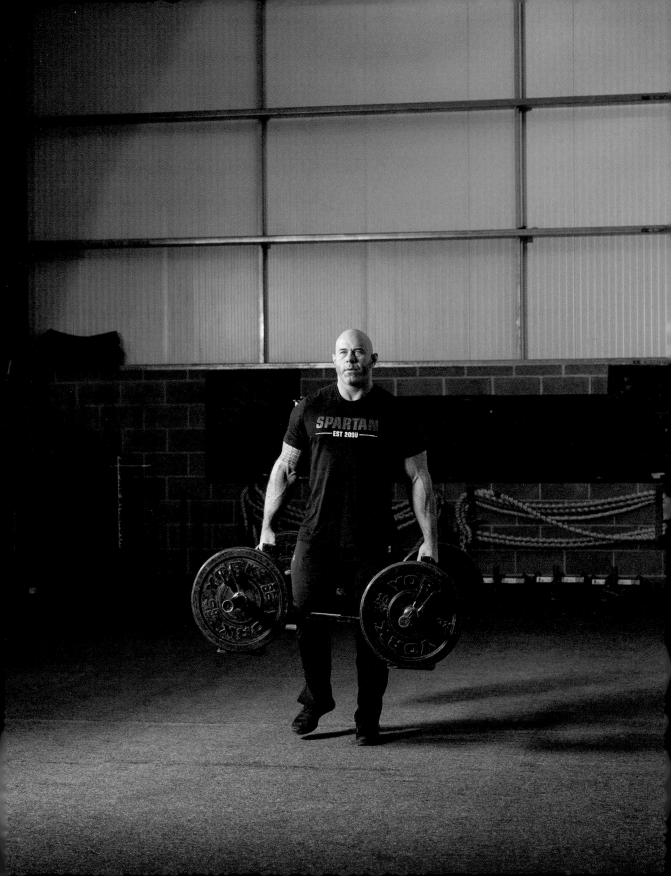

03.

LOADED CARRIES

I've used loaded carries to some degree with nearly every client I have worked with. Their value, in my opinion, is immense. A lot of people associate them with the World's Strongest Man competition and have a preconception that they are just for strongmen or that they need to be performed in the same way that you see the athletes do them on WSM. Of course, they are a great strongman event but they have been shown, thanks to the research of Dr Stuart McGill, to be fantastic for everyday spinal health. What I love about them is that they're simple to perform and easy to coach, and they enhance five key training qualities. And that goes for everyone, not just the strongman population. Here is an overview of why I think they are so useful.

CORE BENEFITS

Any loaded carry demands a strong core brace to protect against both shearing and compressive forces. In doing so they have a profound impact on your performance in the main gym lifts. A strong core is never a weakness. Anyone with a 'soft' midsection during squats, deadlift and overhead presses can be cured with a healthy dose of loaded carries.

What's particularly special to me is that you don't really have to think about said core brace, it just happens. For example, load up a log or axle Zercher carry and perform a set. The very nature and challenge of the exercise itself dictates an automatic core brace regardless of your conscious intent.

INCREASED AWARENESS

You also get enhanced proprioception because you're moving while under load and that's an extremely valuable quality to develop, athlete or not. When I'm coaching someone to do a loaded carry, I don't want them to behave as if they are idly carrying a couple of shopping bags through a supermarket. I require them to secure a brace, and maintain said brace as tight as possible while holding onto the implement and moving under control with purpose. I want my clients fully engaged – no autopilot or going through the motions – in order to maximise the training effect.

MENTAL STRENGTH

Loaded carries not only promote full-body strength, they also develop one of the most important and, in my experience, most overlooked training qualities – mental strength. They may be easy to learn, but whether you are moving a lighter load for long distance or a challenging load for short distance, at some point your mental toughness will be tested.

The farmer's walk, for example, subjects the forearms to a unique level of discomfort. It is easier to put them down a few meters short than go through the pain barrier and complete your distance. Thus they become a valuable diagnostic tool. If someone doesn't complete the specified distance it may be a case of them choosing not to rather than not being able to. Physically they could have done it, but mentally they were not willing to endure that much discomfort.

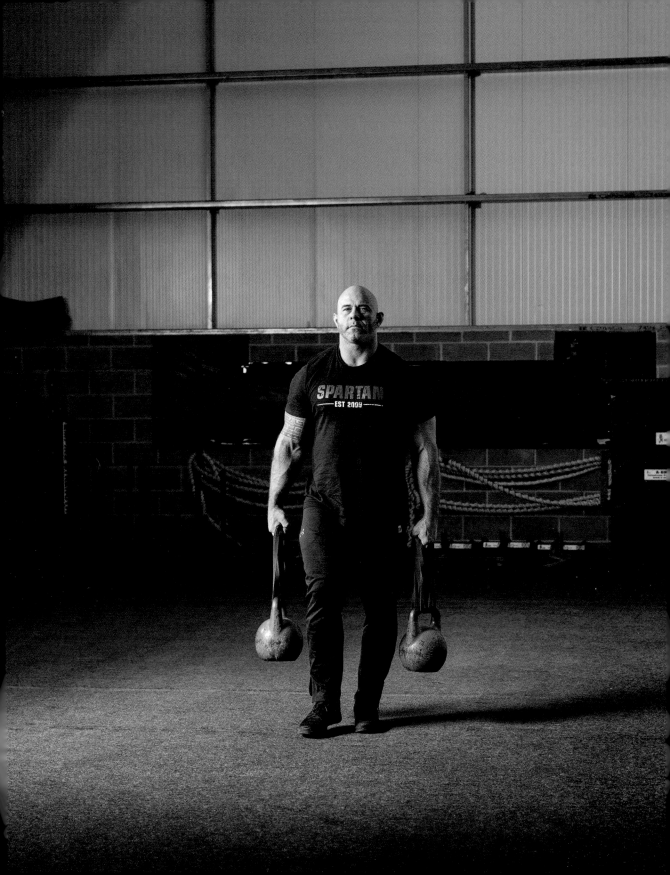

'Loaded carries offer a unique conditioning and fat burning effect. They are my personal choice if someone needs to drop body fat fast'

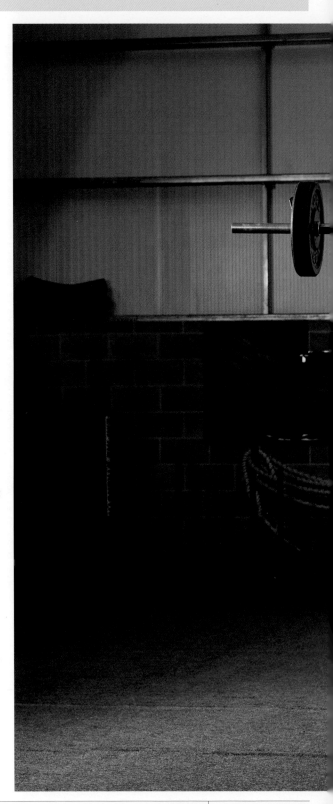

Ultimately, if you want to achieve your strength training potential then you have to go through some level of physical and mental discomfort. In my experience those that endure a suitably weighted loaded carry achieve their goals; those that don't never come close.

MORE MUSCLE

Loaded carries induce hypertrophy in all the right areas thanks to the extended period of muscular tension your body is under when performing them. An appropriately loaded carry is going to require a sustained high level of force output from all musculature to complete. 'Appropriately loaded' being the key concept. I'm not trying to break anyone's body here.

But if you want to get stronger then you're going to have to lift a weight that, for you, is heavy. The key areas that develop are the upper back, forearms and quads. Increased VMO development in your quads, for example, is important for knee stability. Increased upper back strength will certainly aid pressing performance too. I've had lots of guys come into my gym who can bench press decent weight but their upper back is so underdeveloped that at some point its going to become a limiting factor in their strength development.

CONDITIONING TOOL

Loaded carries also offer a unique conditioning and fat burning effect. They are my personal choice if someone needs to drop body fat fast. They offer a huge bang for your buck here.

Even if you perform a carry on its own you will still be working the full body at all times, and carrying heavy loads for long durations forces you to work hard and intense. The greater the intensity, the greater the metabolic impact.

However, if you really want to up the fat loss ante, perform them as part of a medley. Combine two or three different loaded carries in a circuit such as farmer's walk into prowler push into Zercher carry. This vastly increases the training density and fat burning effect.

So those are the five key benefits, and we can emphasise any one of them depending on how we programme the loaded carry. What you're looking at is one movement, which is very easy to teach and to implement within a workout, and you've got five valuable qualities that can be enhanced by doing it. That, for me, makes them a no-brainer to include in any strength training programme.

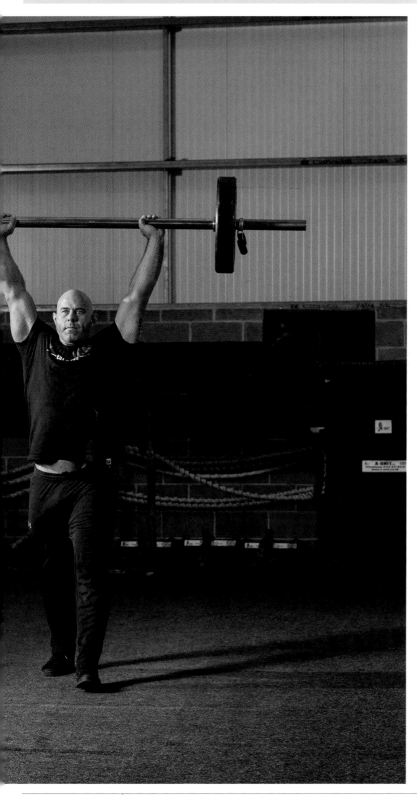

Takeaway tips

THE MORE THE BETTER

I'd incorporate loaded carries into every session or, at a minimum, every week. For me they are not an exercise to cycle into a programme occasionally. They are a regular fixture in my own training and the programmes of all my clients, regardless of their goal, and there aren't many exercises I can say that for. In the best case scenario, you'd do them every session because the return is so high. You get so much value from the exercise in such a short space of time. In my opinion, a workout without a variation of them is lacking. They're not just physically beneficial, they're satisfying to do too, so they keep you engaged in the session.

BE SMART WITH LOADING

For the purposes of this book, I'm more concerned with how you perform loaded carries for the sets and distance as opposed to the load. There are two main ways that you can perform loaded carries. The first is a sprint race, where you cover a distance as quickly as possible and technique becomes secondary to time taken. This is what you see in strongman competitions, and it is valid for that sport. But if you're training for specific strength benefits, I want you to carry the load with a rigid body. I want tension from head to toe and I want you to maintain that tension for the entire distance.

DITCH THE BELT

Ideally I'd want you to perform your loaded carries without the aid of a lifting belt and develop a truly formidable core. This is a strength that will never let you down throughout your lifting journey. Certainly at some point wearing a belt can not only be prudent, but beneficial too, but I'd advise against relying on a belt too soon. It may well see you carry more weight, but I want you to develop your own belt – your core – before your ego.

Farmer's walk progression

These are the four progressive stages I coach my clients through to master the farmer's walk

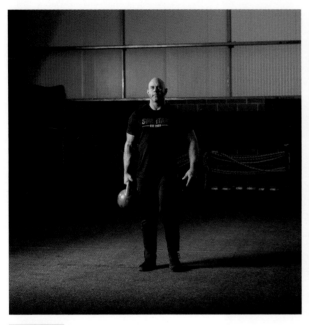

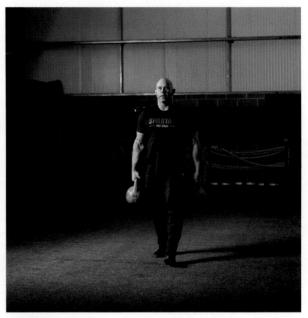

LEVEL 1
Unilateral farmer's walk

I prefer to start with unilateral rather than bilateral because at this stage we're not chasing weight. We're purely focusing on movement mastery and technique. If you start bilaterally, the technique isn't a massive challenge. I like to emphasise the importance of understanding how to brace and maintain a brace, and the unilateral version brings that to the fore, as well as increasing proprioception.

LEVEL 2
Bilateral farmer's walk

The bilateral farmer's walk is arguably the most recognisable loaded carry variation. Once you've mastered the unilateral version you can start loading bilaterally, which will increase the stimulus and training effect.

COACHING MASTERCLASS

When someone is performing the unilateral version a valuable coaching cue is to get them to touch their abs and obliques with their free hand and feel that they are engaged and braced effectively.

I want them to understand exactly how the perfect brace should feel throughout their entire core. Instead of simply responding to my cue to 'brace', the client is instead acutely aware of how their torso should feel when braced – as you can with a unilateral farmer's walk – then they can understand and apply it so much easier. Crucially, when I talk about a brace I'm talking about real intra-abdominal pressure, which actually means your abs will be pushed out, not sucked in as if you were posing for a photograph.

Finally, the unilateral version instils increased discipline and focus because it presents more of a technical challenge than the bilateral version, and I'd prefer to drill those qualities early on and emphasise the importance of quality over weight.

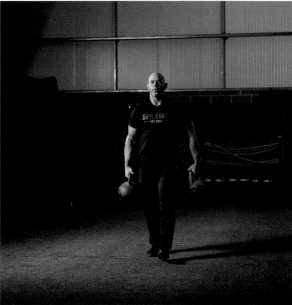

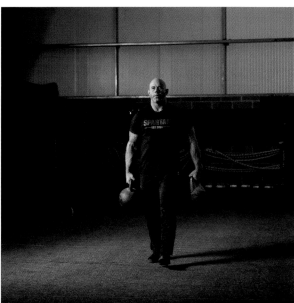

LEVEL 3
Uneven load farmer's walk

You could just keep adding weight to the bilateral farmer's walk, but I like to milk as much as possible from a specific load before increasing it, and an uneven load allows you to do that. The beauty of this move is that you can maintain or even reduce the total load carried but you increase the core engagement. Just make sure you do an equal amount of sets on both sides. The uneven version is also useful if you don't have access to really heavy dumbbells because it requires lighter loads than the bilateral farmer's walk to get the desired training effect.

LEVEL 4
Hanging band technique

Hanging band technique (HBT) is the icing on the training cake, whether that's for carries or barbell work. If you master the basics, you then have the option of progressing to HBT for extra stimulus. Requiring increased grip strength, endurance, coordination and skill to perform effectively, this is not for everyone – I find HBT to be most suitable for more experienced individuals. Just because you can do it doesn't mean you necessarily should. No one client uses every bit of kit that I have. As a coach I urge you to choose your tools wisely on an individual basis.

Level 1
Unilateral farmer's walk

WHY

The key element of this variation is that the abdominals have to work in a way that's anti-rotational, which is an important quality to develop. You don't just want to train the abdominals by flexing all the time. When you have a weight in one hand your body wants to twist or fall over to that side so you have to stabilise. I'd say this is a more challenging version than the bilateral farmer's walk that we covered in the foundation chapter (p56) because you really have to focus on what you're doing. You won't use as heavy a load but that's another important factor. Whenever I coach someone I'm always trying to get as much out of an exercise or a weight as I can before I increase the load. The longer I've been coaching, the more value I see in getting as much out of a weight as possible before moving on.

HOW

I always start people by using one weight on one side but I cue them to imagine that they are holding two weights. Begin by hinging down as if you were going to perform a trap bar deadlift. Imagine that you're grabbing a weight on both sides – as if we've Photoshopped the second weight out of the picture.

Grip the weight and brace your entire core. It shouldn't look like you're being pulled over to one side because we want the other side to fire and stabilise too. This is a great drill to use to reinforce bracing mechanics, which is a key point that I keep coming back to. So deadlift the weight to standing, pause and re-brace. Your aim once you start walking is to move the weight over the desired distance while staying as rigid as possible.

The challenge isn't so much moving the weight, it's how you move the weight – how well you brace, maintain that brace and maintain that core rigidity. I want your movement to be steady and controlled, and I want your torso to be bulletproof as a result.

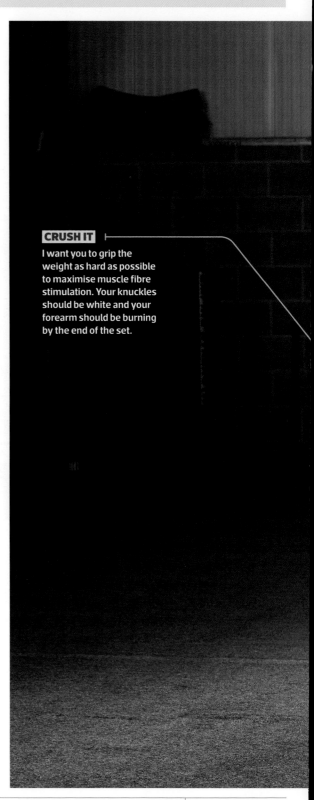

CRUSH IT

I want you to grip the weight as hard as possible to maximise muscle fibre stimulation. Your knuckles should be white and your forearm should be burning by the end of the set.

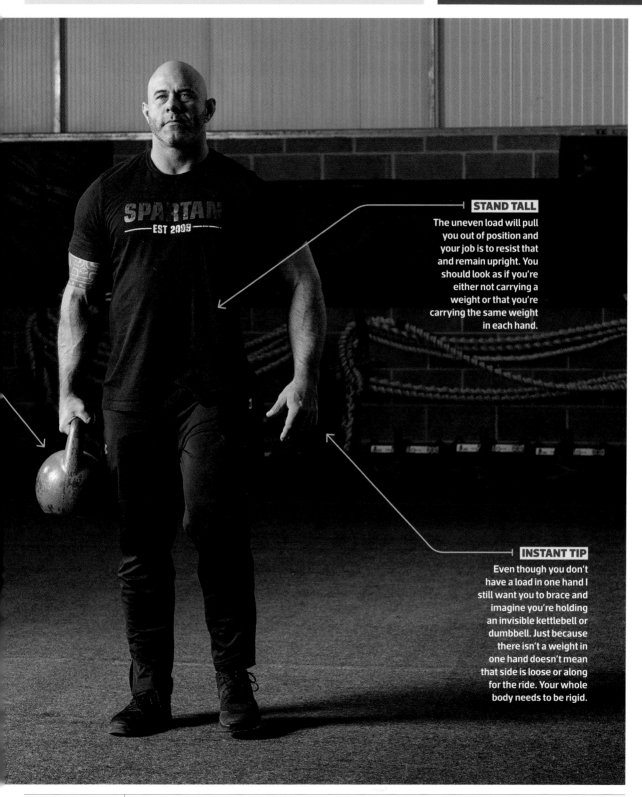

STAND TALL

The uneven load will pull you out of position and your job is to resist that and remain upright. You should look as if you're either not carrying a weight or that you're carrying the same weight in each hand.

INSTANT TIP

Even though you don't have a load in one hand I still want you to brace and imagine you're holding an invisible kettlebell or dumbbell. Just because there isn't a weight in one hand doesn't mean that side is loose or along for the ride. Your whole body needs to be rigid.

Level 2
Bilateral farmer's walk

WHY

We start the farmer's walk progression with the unilateral version to make sure that your abdominals and core are switched on. Once you progress from that it's time to get an even load in each hand. That gives you significant scope for progression because as you get stronger, the load you carry gets heavier – provided you maintain good form.

HOW

The pick-up technique is the same as in the unilateral version, only this time you really do have a weight in each hand. It might be useful to think that you're hinging to pick up the weights by the side of your body as if you were doing a trap bar deadlift. You should already be proficient in bracing with one weight, and both the coaching cues and the movement are the same as with the unilateral version.

Again, I want to see a steady pace with a rigid body. As your ability to brace increases we can increase the pace of the carry, which will be done by taking quicker not bigger steps – but never at the expense of the brace.

If you're turning while holding the weight then your turns should be slow and controlled. Decelerate, pause, turn carefully, pause again and re-brace before starting the return leg. I always get people to imagine that they are carrying two full buckets of water and that they are trying not to spill a drop.

At the finish, you want to pause, come to a dead stop and hinge to lower the weights under control. That may not seem important but I value the mental toughness and discipline that finishing the move properly brings. No matter how tired your grip is, I always want you to be in control of the weight.

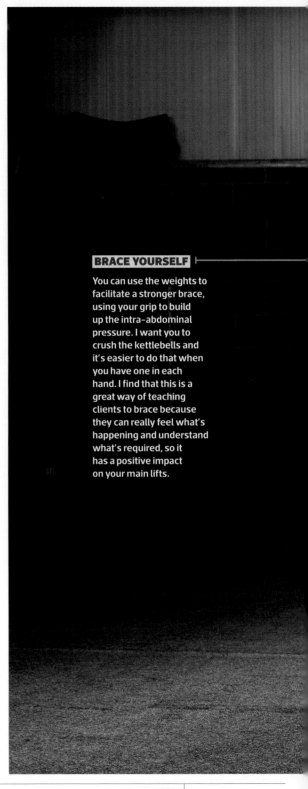

BRACE YOURSELF

You can use the weights to facilitate a stronger brace, using your grip to build up the intra-abdominal pressure. I want you to crush the kettlebells and it's easier to do that when you have one in each hand. I find that this is a great way of teaching clients to brace because they can really feel what's happening and understand what's required, so it has a positive impact on your main lifts.

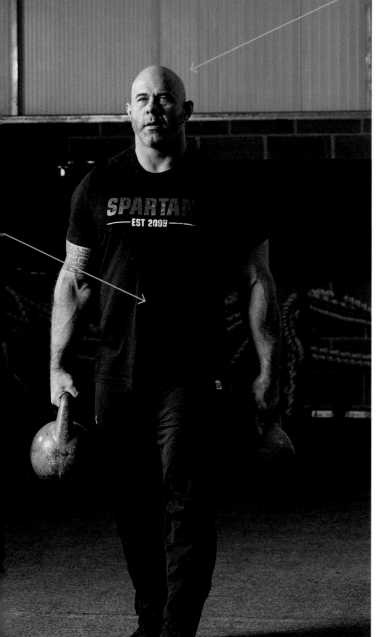

EYES FRONT

I want tunnel vision, not looking at the floor or to the side. Your gaze should be fixed on the horizon. Turning your head signals a lack of application and opens a weak link in the chain. I want your body to be as rigid as possible. The only moving parts should be the legs.

PROGRESSION
Farmer's frame

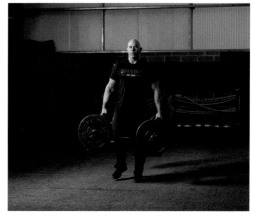

If the aim is to move as much weight as possible, I use a farmer's walk frame. The grips are quite wide apart – wider than a trap bar – so you get a greater emphasis on grip strength and back strength when you pick it up. The benefit of the frame is that it gives you more space for your legs so it won't impede your stride pattern. You can do farmer's walks with a trap bar frame and even those soft square frames I've seen in health clubs. The handles on those tend to be made of rope, which poses an even greater grip strength challenge.

When we're talking about going heavy, as on this move, it's worth pointing out that I prefer doing farmer's walks without a lifting belt because a belt will negate the core benefits. We only use belts with heavier loads in strongman training where speed is important. But for establishing a good strength foundation, I'd rather focus on maintaining a brace position for a sustained period of time without the aid of a belt.

Level 3
Uneven load farmer's walk

WHY

The aim here is to train your body to stabilise. It's also rather forgiving on your central nervous system (CNS). If you always lift heavy it will be physically and mentally draining so it's about being smart with your loading parameters. It doesn't mean you can't build up the weight over time but it took me a long time to realise that more isn't always better. If you asked me a few years ago I might have said, 'more, more, more' but now I realise the power of using the minimum effective dose.

If you want to play around with this move you can look at the thickness of the handle. You can either use normal or fat grips. You can easily attach a fat grip handle to a dumbbell if you train in a commercial gym and that will make it more of a grip test rather than an anti-rotation move.

This is also a good warm-up for a heavy farmer's walk or a deadlift session. The extra challenge presented by the uneven load forces you to really focus because it can catch you off-guard. I like my clients to be in tune with what they are doing because it will have a positive carryover to everything else you do in the gym. I don't really like absolutes and I usually say 'that depends' when it comes to questions about training, but this is as close to an absolute as I get – the importance of the ability to brace and maintain a brace during lifts and carries is essential.

HOW MUCH

You don't have to go heavy. If you can lift two 30kg dumbbells in a bilateral farmer's walk you could lift one 30kg dumbbell and one 15kg dumbbell for an uneven farmer's walk. To give you a bit of context, if I'm training for a strongman competition I might lift 150-160kg in each hand for a bilateral farmer's walk. But for this variation I might use a 50kg and a 28kg kettlebell. Not an enormous load, but that's not the point.

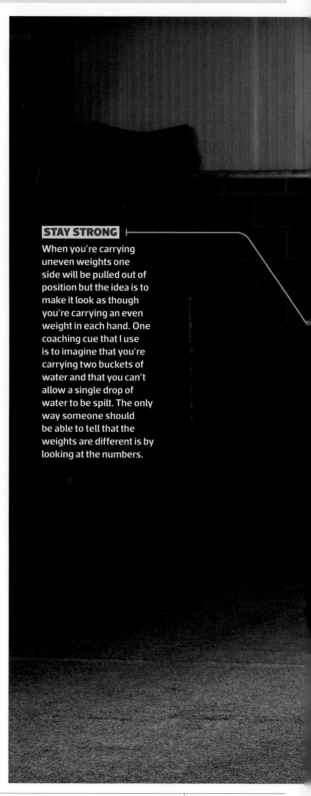

STAY STRONG

When you're carrying uneven weights one side will be pulled out of position but the idea is to make it look as though you're carrying an even weight in each hand. One coaching cue that I use is to imagine that you're carrying two buckets of water and that you can't allow a single drop of water to be spilt. The only way someone should be able to tell that the weights are different is by looking at the numbers.

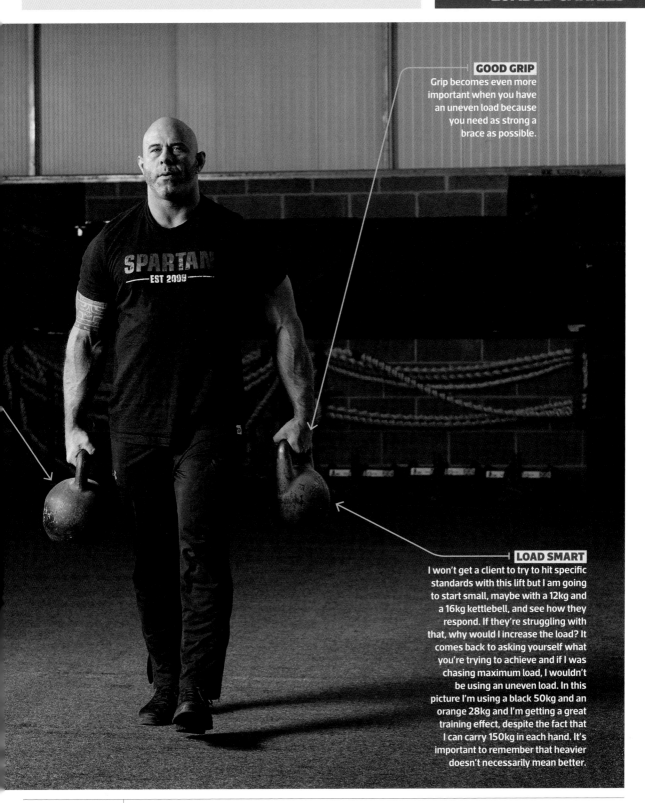

GOOD GRIP

Grip becomes even more important when you have an uneven load because you need as strong a brace as possible.

LOAD SMART

I won't get a client to try to hit specific standards with this lift but I am going to start small, maybe with a 12kg and a 16kg kettlebell, and see how they respond. If they're struggling with that, why would I increase the load? It comes back to asking yourself what you're trying to achieve and if I was chasing maximum load, I wouldn't be using an uneven load. In this picture I'm using a black 50kg and an orange 28kg and I'm getting a great training effect, despite the fact that I can carry 150kg in each hand. It's important to remember that heavier doesn't necessarily mean better.

Level 4
Hanging band technique

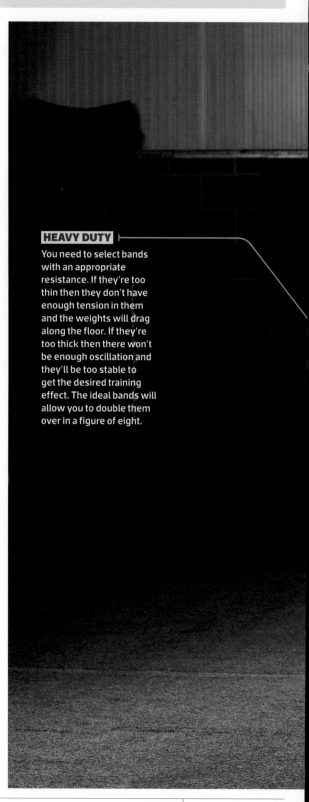

You need to select bands with an appropriate resistance. If they're too thin then they don't have enough tension in them and the weights will drag along the floor. If they're too thick then there won't be enough oscillation and they'll be too stable to get the desired training effect. The ideal bands will allow you to double them over in a figure of eight.

WHY

For the HBT version you take bands, loop them around the horns of a kettlebell, and hold them in your hands. Bands are tough to grip. You get the benefits of a conventional farmer's walk but with the hanging bands the weights will bounce around so you require greater neuromuscular coordination to stabilise them which, in turn, will result in increased motor unit recruitment. Sure, it looks cool but there's a solid theory behind it as well. You also get increased intra-muscular and inter-muscular coordination.

Even better, you get all that without even having to think about it. You don't consciously think, 'Right, I'm going to try to increase my intra-muscular coordination' – it just happens. That, as far as I'm concerned, makes it an efficient exercise because I can get a lot of benefits with as few coaching cues as possible. The bands will also have a positive effect on your overall farmer's walk technique because it will teach you to tighten your core and engage muscles all over your body. That will have a hypertrophy benefit too. You've got to maintain constant tension and get as tight as hell. You can't relax so that means your time under tension goes up.

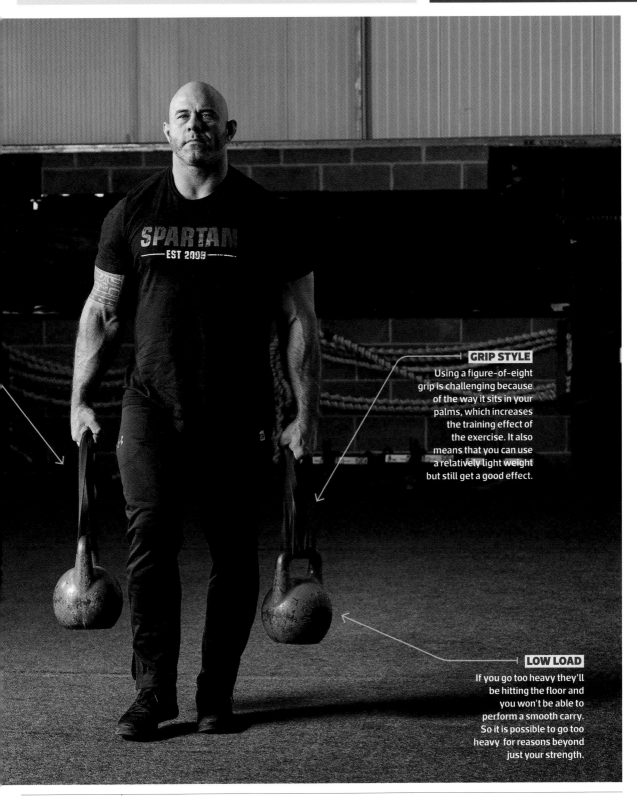

GRIP STYLE

Using a figure-of-eight grip is challenging because of the way it sits in your palms, which increases the training effect of the exercise. It also means that you can use a relatively light weight but still get a good effect.

LOW LOAD

If you go too heavy they'll be hitting the floor and you won't be able to perform a smooth carry. So it is possible to go too heavy for reasons beyond just your strength.

Zercher carry

WHY

This is my personal favourite core exercise. It has a certain visual appeal and I'm drawn to that sort of exercise. It's a bit like a big tyre being flipped – it just carries extra kudos. But it's not just about how it looks. When the weight is in front of your body, that requires enormous core recruitment. And when I talk about the core I'm talking about all the muscles between the neck and the knees – front, back and sides – not just the six or eight visible abs that may look pretty if your body fat is low enough.

I find that the Zercher carry is very good at teaching people to breathe and brace simultaneously. You can do a farmer's walk without bracing properly but it is much harder to do a Zercher carry without bracing, which is one of the reasons I like it.

I prefer to use a log rather than a barbell because a thin bar limits you from a pain perspective and you can't carry the load or go the distance that's required to get the training effect. An added bonus is that logs have a greater diameter so the centre of gravity is further away from your body, which will increase the stress on your core musculature. You get increased upper back emphasis and a huge biceps and forearm pump too, while your delts are stimulated and your pecs are on fire. It also looks fucking awesome and is a core destroyer. There's no way you can perform it correctly and not feel it. I prefer to take the load out of two squat stands rather than trying to pick it up off the floor but you could also take it out of a power rack or lift it off boxes.

HOW

To lift it out of squat stands it's essentially a ¼ Zercher squat to lock-out. Aim to carry the weight as high up your chest as possible rather than at your navel because carrying it low will force you to round your back, which we don't want. When the weight is higher you get better core engagement and your upper back works harder to maintain this position.

I want you to use the same approach as the farmer's walk – slow and controlled steps. The key thing to focus on is the tension you create and maintain in the midsection. The quality of the carry, not the weight that you're lifting, is what is most important. Again, take quicker, not longer, steps as you progress. If you take bigger steps then you will lose stability from the legs and your brace will be compromised.

CHEST IS BEST

I don't want to see the load below sternum height. It should be high on your chest, pulled in to your body and held as firmly as possible. Just as we want your knuckles turning white on a bilateral carry, we want your upper back rigid, your core braced and tension in your arms.

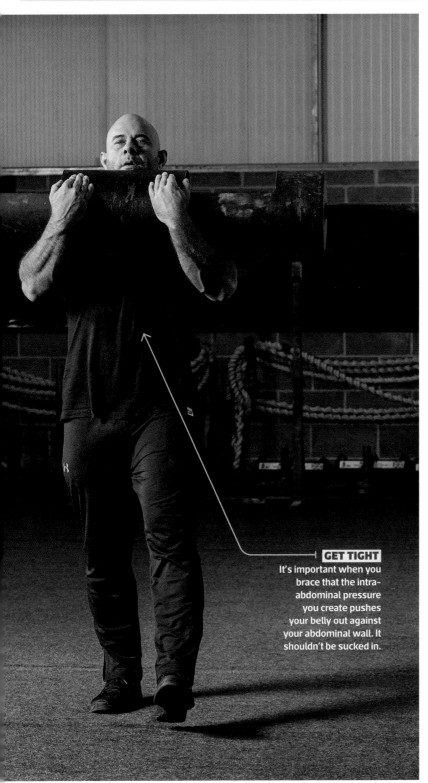

GET TIGHT
It's important when you brace that the intra-abdominal pressure you create pushes your belly out against your abdominal wall. It shouldn't be sucked in.

PROGRESSION
Zercher hanging band

The only progression for the Zercher carry I use is with the addition of hanging bands. First you master the main lift, then you build the weight, and then you can use bands. But that only applies to a select group of trainees.

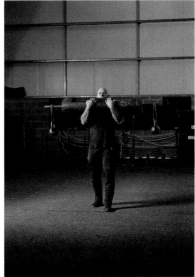

GEAR UPGRADE

Some gyms have a strongman yoke that looks a bit like a squat stand. That can be adjusted to do a Zercher carry. These are good because you can easily adjust the crossbar to the optimal pick-up height for different individuals. The crossbars tend to be thick too which is never a bad thing.

Overhead carry

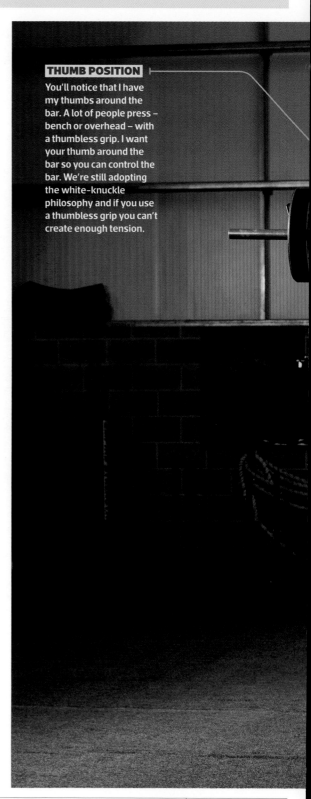

WHY

I've always taken training inspiration from the greats of the past. Legends such as Fred Hatfield, Bill Kazmaier, George Hackenschmidt, Ed Coan and Paul Anderson. It was the training of world champion weightlifter Vasily Alekseyev that first brought overhead carries to my attention.

They are great for developing shoulder stability, as well as your obliques and serratus muscles. They will also develop your traps and triceps and are superb for improving lock-out strength in the bench and overhead press. I love doing them and always feel stronger and more powerful when they are in my programme.

Despite my love for this lift, I do not use it with all clients, simply because not everyone has the flexibility and mobility to perform it safely. This is often because they have tight pecs and lats so they'll overcompensate by hyperextending the lower back. If I am going to use it I'll only do so if I can be sure that they can get into the loaded position correctly.

HOW

You want to press the weight overhead and then shrug your traps up – like you're trying to push the weight through the ceiling. That gives you greater upper back stimulus and development. Grip the bar as tightly as possible and imagine trying to pull it apart. It's vital that you secure the perfect lock-out before you start to move. I find that it is usually a lack of endurance in the triceps and upper back that limits people, so always start light and progress slowly. A little can go a long way on this exercise.

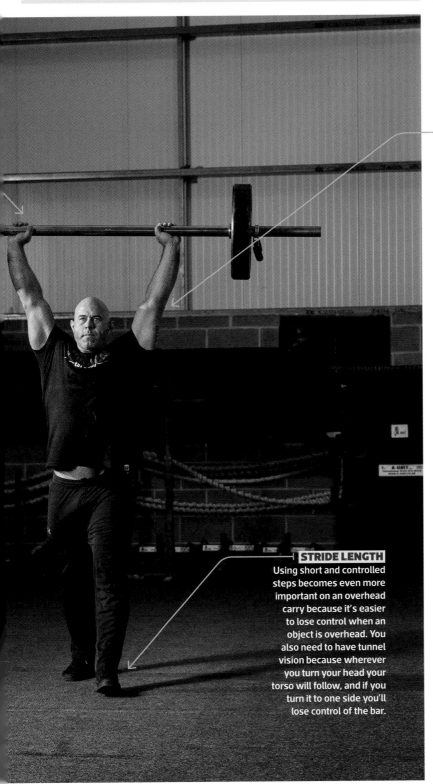

LOCK OUT

You should shrug your traps up and try to press the bar through the ceiling at all times to really engage the upper back musculature. I also want you to grip the bar hard and try to pull it apart to get the biggest possible training effect.

STRIDE LENGTH

Using short and controlled steps becomes even more important on an overhead carry because it's easier to lose control when an object is overhead. You also need to have tunnel vision because wherever you turn your head your torso will follow, and if you turn it to one side you'll lose control of the bar.

PROGRESSIONS

Simply start with an empty bar and progress by adding load. There are so many variations: you can use a bar, a log, dumbbells or even kettlebells. I find dumbbells can be kinder on the shoulder and elbow joints because the barbell grip is fixed, whereas they are not. Having said that, my preference is to use a barbell because you can easily add load and increase the training effect.

Logs are particularly good for combat and throwing athletes because they can use a neutral grip which is kinder on their wrists, elbows and shoulders. The thicker diameter of the log requires a greater core emphasis to balance overhead too.

Once you've mastered those you could move on to employing the hanging band technique. Very little will light up your core, shoulders and triceps like the HBT on this exercise, but this will probably only be appropriate for a small number of people. It is vital that you choose the right tool for the individual.

Loading parameters

Here's how to adapt your loaded carry training variables to match your training goal

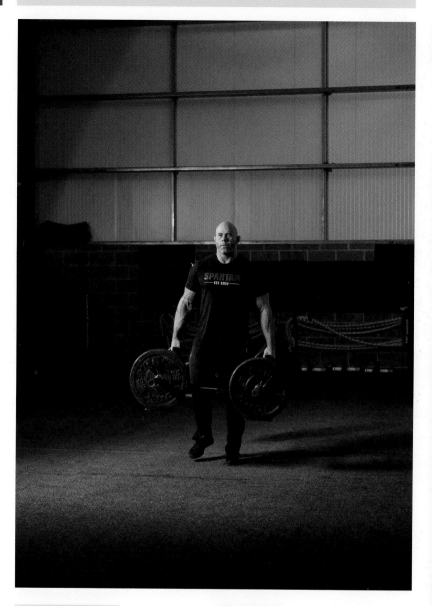

STRENGTH

MINIMUM DISTANCE 10m
MAXIMUM DISTANCE 60m
IDEAL DISTANCE 20-40m

In my view, less than 10m will offer very little training effect. There's always a minimum amount of work in order to gain a suitable return. For example, when training barbell lifts for strength, I might do 3-5 reps but I wouldn't do half a rep. These parameters are based on my own experience and the space that I have at my gym.

1-3 warm-up sets
3-5 work sets
2-3min rest between sets
1 set is a set distance

EFFORT AND INTENSITY
This should be the same as if you were doing a barbell lift of five sets of five reps. The last set should be a five-rep max, which means you should be able to perform five reps perfectly but no more. I want you to use as much weight as possible but I don't want you crashing over the line. I want you to finish under control while being at your limit.

HYPERTROPHY

MINIMUM DISTANCE 40m
MAXIMUM DISTANCE 80m
IDEAL DISTANCE 60m
The aim with hypertrophy is to increase the time under tension compared with strength work but not so much that it becomes an endurance test.

1-3 warm-up sets
3-5 work sets
90sec-2min rest between sets

FAT LOSS

You can either carry for distance, 60-100m, or for time, 60-90 seconds with a weight in hand. But it's not an exact science. For fat loss I like to maximise time under tension while seeing rest periods incomplete.

4-6 sets
60-90sec rest
Or a 1:1 work:rest ratio

Programming loaded carries

How to start incorporating carries into your training plan

Using carries in a session

Loaded carries can turn into a medley or you can superset them. For example:

A1. **40m FARMER'S WALK**
A2. **40m ZERCHER CARRY**
A3. **40m OVERHEAD CARRY**

You can also use sled pulls and prowler pushes with carries – in fact, I highly recommend this approach. In doing so a medley could look like this:

A1. **20m FARMER'S WALK**
A2. **20m PROWLER PUSH**
A3. **20m BACKWARD SLED PULL**

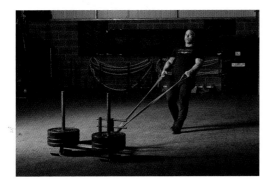

In the foundation phase a loaded carry can be performed as part of every workout in the form of either a farmer's walk, prowler push or sled pull. I'd probably do a variation in every session and you can cycle through your options. At this stage I like to build as broad and solid a foundation as possible.

If you're training the key barbell lifts, I'd at least have a loaded carry on lower body days. You could perform a farmer's walk on deadlift day and a Zercher carry on squat day. But you could also do the reverse and the results would be very similar. Quite often at this stage it is dictated by the ability of the individual. As valuable as they are, loaded carries can be very taxing on the body.

Sample four-day split

SESSION 1
DEADLIFT AND FARMER'S WALK

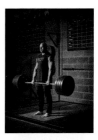

SESSION 2
SQUAT AND ZERCHER CARRY

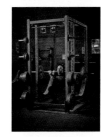

SESSION 3
OVERHEAD PRESS AND OVERHEAD CARRY

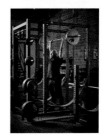

SESSION 4
BENCH PRESS AND PROWLER PUSH

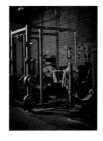

How you use loaded carries depends on the person. The question I'd ask is what's the maximum volume you can reasonably handle during the session? Also, can you recover? After all, it doesn't matter how many bullet-point benefits an exercise has if you can't perform it properly or aren't ready to train.

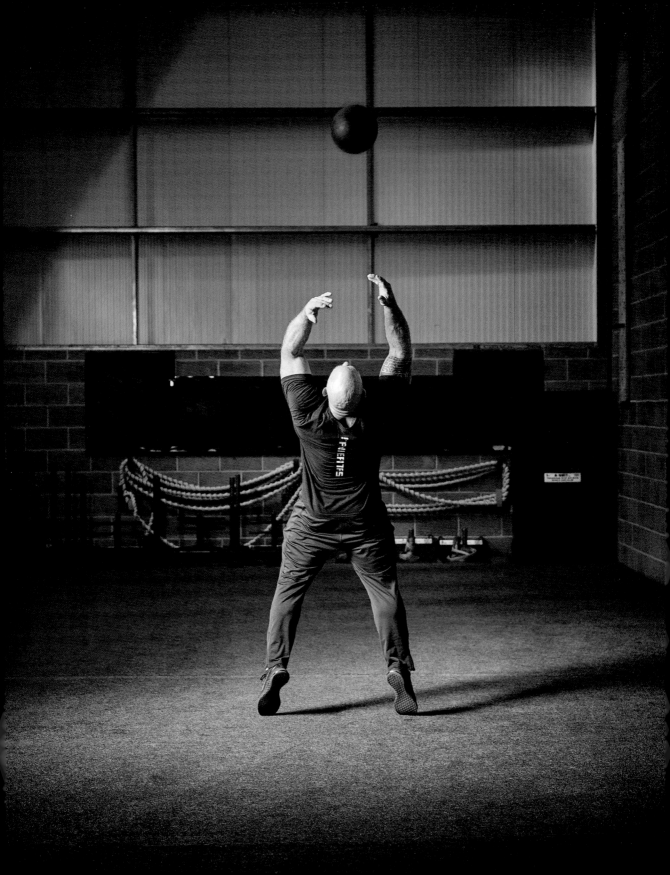

04.

POWER TRAINING

By developing a client's power I can make a positive impact on their strength development and vice versa. Powerful individuals are able to generate more force and display their strength quicker than those less powerful by demonstrating a higher rate of force development.

Before I incorporate specific power training exercises, though, I first have all my clients make the most of the main barbell lifts to develop maximal strength. They are my number one way to develop strength and power. For less experienced individuals, any increase in maximum strength will also lead to an increase in power so I focus on those first and foremost. Save as many tools and tricks for down the line as you can. The more advanced you become, the tougher results become to attain.

NERVOUS ENERGY

Power movements are, for me, the ultimate pre-workout cocktail and you can't buy it by the scoop. Your CNS sends commands to your muscles and we want that message to get there as quickly and efficiently as possible. I like to do so simply and use exercises that are easy to teach and implement, such as jumping rope and med ball slams. These help excite the nervous system and ensure a productive session ensues.

Most people have significant work and life commitments to fit around their workouts, and sometimes the last thing that they feel like doing is training. One of a coach's biggest responsibilities is to change that. Once you've done the sensible stuff – increased blood flow and muscle pliability at the start of their warm-up – power drills can get people fired up for a productive session.

Studies have also shown that the correct power drills can also improve your strength training performance within a session. For example, researchers have shown that when subjects did box jumps before squats, their squat performance was improved compared with those who didn't do the jumps.

UNLEASH YOUR INNER ATHLETE

Initially we use power drills just to excite the CNS. But ultimately you're going to develop an appreciable level of strength across the barbell lifts. In which case, your continued progression will benefit from an increase in rate of force development. That's very much how I train athletes, and I've deliberately tried to keep that out of the equation in this book because it's about general strength training, not elite athlete training.

For athletes, power drills are an integral part of their training. It can be the game-changer. On the sporting field you'll find two types of people. The skinny dude who is lightning fast but if he runs into someone he falls to pieces. Well, that's not much use. Or you've got a huge fucker who can squat the world but he can't get out of the way of his own shadow. That's not much use on the sports field either, is it? What we're looking for in true athletic development is the magic combination of both strength and speed. We want a powerful athlete.

These drills will give you an insight into that kind of training. We want to do something fast and aggressive so jumps and throws are great. We're also aiming to make the workout as productive as possible. The drill should also be specific to the person training. The more advanced they are, the more advanced the drill can be. Having said that, even when I'm training elite athletes I try to make the drills as simple as possible. The reason I've chosen the exercises in this chapter is because they are the easiest to teach and learn. As I said, many people's training time is scarce and precious, so you want to maximise the return.

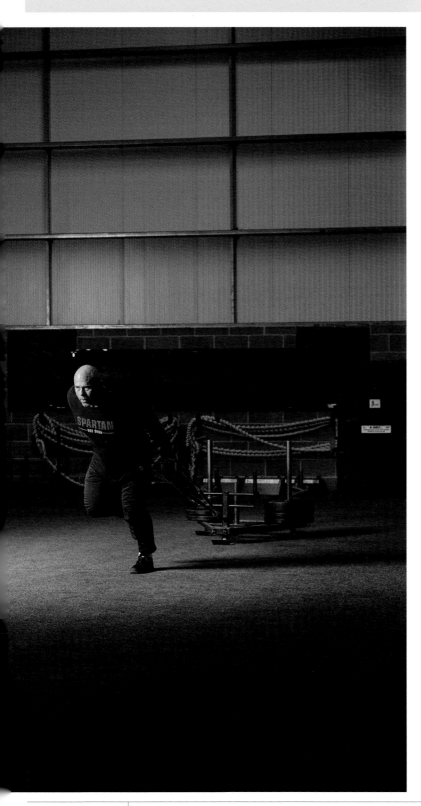

Takeaway tips

GO ALL-OUT

I want you to devote maximum application to every rep you perform. I like the phrase that Mike Tyson used to describe his training. He hit the bag with 'bad intentions' and I want you to use that same intensity. You can't just go through the motions and I never want to see a half-arsed box jump. It's a mindset thing that you have to adopt if you want to get the most out of the moves in this chapter. Every rep needs to be explosive. So if you're doing a medicine ball slam, for example, I don't want you to just drop it to the floor. I want you to throw it through the floor. When you do a box jump I want you to try to jump through the ceiling.

ONLY PERFORM GOOD-QUALITY REPS

Just because I'm asking you to be violent in your execution, that isn't an excuse to be sloppy. So when the speed of execution decreases, the set stops. When I programme these exercises I'll typically get clients to do 3-5 reps, which encourages quality of execution. If someone is new to power development training we need to keep their reps as low as possible to maintain speed. Remember, I'd always take two superb reps over four good ones. And these moves aren't about going heavy. It's all about the execution.

RECOVER FULLY BETWEEN SETS

When you're training for power development you must rest fully between sets. You want to exert 100% power output each set because we're using these movements to excite the CNS and to increase your rate of force development. Exercises such as box jumps and med ball slams are often associated with metabolic conditioning workouts that are typically high-rep, low-skill and done under fatigue. That's not what we're doing here, we're approaching things from a totally different perspective, so make sure that you recover properly between sets.

Jumping rope

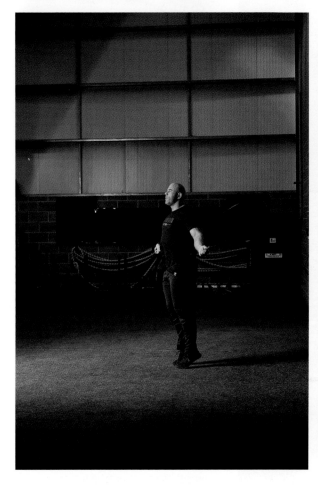

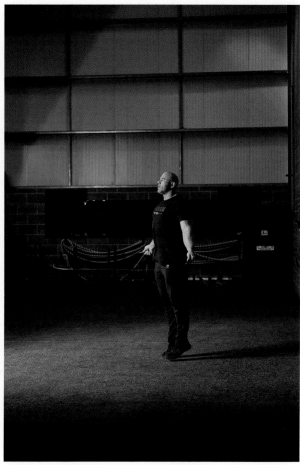

You can use rope jumping as a base plyometric. It's easy to set up and learn, and it offers multiple benefits.

Generally overlooked outside fight sports, simple rope jumping will fire up your nervous system while increasing athleticism, coordination and core musculature temperature. It also helps condition your lower body for explosive activity and offers a hell of a fitness boost while presenting a low risk of injury.

You can make skipping as simple or as complicated as you want but you don't have to impersonate a *Rocky* montage to benefit. Just focus on finding your rhythm and being light on your feet. I like to keep it simple. In CrossFit they'll do double-unders and triple-unders which are great but I don't expect them. As long as the rope goes over your head and under your feet, I'm happy.

FORM

I want you to be as relaxed as possible and I want you to jump just high enough so that the rope goes under your feet and over your head. As you progress you can bring your arms into it more. The rope will go faster so you have to react faster and it becomes more demanding.

LOAD

- Start with 5 sets of 30sec with a 1:1 work:rest ratio.
- Build up to doing 5 sets of 60sec with a 1:1 work:rest ratio.
- I find both of the above protocols to be a simple and effective way to provide a training stimulus without being too taxing. If you're a fighter you may build up to 3-5 minutes unbroken. My advice is to apply it on an individual basis.

Box jump

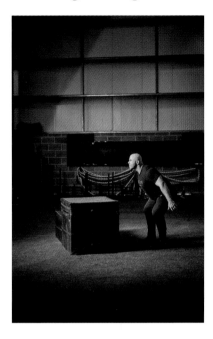
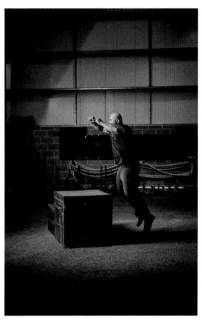
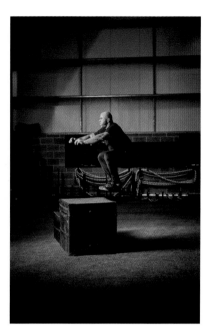

If you want a great lower body power drill, I'd go for box jumps. Jumps are the best way to develop explosive strength for lifting. I prefer to use the soft plyo boxes that are widely available. The old-school wooden ones are cheaper and have a certain raw appeal, but if you hit your shins on them then it's game over as far as focus goes. Inevitably clients end up too concerned with avoiding injury and that compromises jump performance.

Soft plyo boxes also decrease joint stress and provide a surface that is great to develop correct landing mechanics. While most clients are able to jump, very few know how to land correctly. Doing so while exhibiting proper body control is crucial to safe and effective jump training. Imagine a Bugatti – it's an amazing supercar but if the brakes aren't working then it's an accident waiting to happen. It's actually quite rare for me to come across an individual who knows how to land without being coached. I often see people landing very heavy, knees collapsing inwards and tipping forwards onto their toes.

The most common mistake that I see from coaches is trying to get their clients to jump as high as possible. Don't worry, I did too once. I had a Premier League footballer hitting 54in [137cm] box jumps with relative ease. Sure they looked impressive, but in reality I was taking needless risk exhibiting his excellent hip flexibility instead of focusing on maximising his power development. As a coach you need to be clear not only what you want an exercise to achieve but also exactly how you will execute it in order to effectively achieve your goal.

FORM

Think of this as a full-body exercise. It's not just your legs working – your arms are massively involved too, contributing up to 10% towards jump performance. Start by descending into a shallow squat, arms back as you load the glutes and hamstrings, then explode up through the legs onto the box. When you go into triple extension and leave the floor, your arms should lead the way to give you added momentum. Land solidly, shoulders in front of the knees, your feet roughly shoulder-width apart in an athletic stance – a quarter squat position.

LOAD

- Box jumps should be exclusively reserved for the end of a thorough warm-up where you can focus on increasing rate of force development and exciting the CNS while fresh. The quality of each jump is crucial, as is complete rest between sets. I'm not using them as part of a metabolic conditioning circuit.
- Do 3-5 sets of 3-5 reps.
- Rest until you have recovered completely and go again.
- If you do more volume than that, you'll probably find the quality will diminish.

Slam ball slam

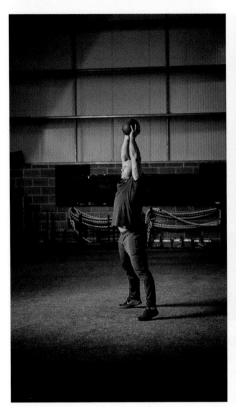
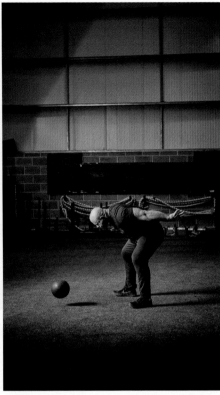

COACHING INSIGHT

TRIPLE THREAT

I want you to focus on triple extension so that you extend your arms above your head when you're on your tiptoes. There are two ways of doing that. The correct way is to reach straight up to the ceiling. I don't want you to move your arms behind your head as if you were taking a soccer throw-in. We want you to reach up and slam down, not backwards then forwards and down.

HIP ACTION

The majority of the movement is at the hips so it is similar to a Russian kettlebell swing. When you throw the ball, the hips hinge backwards to bring in your glutes and hamstrings. Your aim, as with all power-based exercises, should be to slam down as violently as possible.

QUALITY COUNTS

I'm always looking for quality of slam. When I'm coaching people I cue them to execute power moves with 'bad intentions'. It's how it hits the floor that matters. I can tell how well a client is doing without looking at them because you can hear the sound of the impact and judge the quality of the rep by the sound that it makes.

I'd generally use this before a training session that was hip-hinge focused, such as a deadlift workout. You simply reach as high as you can to go into full triple extension, then slam the ball down with as much force as possible. It's easy to teach and you can quantify the quality of the rep. You don't even have to look – you can hear the quality by the sound the ball makes when it hits the floor. You're trying to throw the ball through the floor so slam it as hard as possible.

Another reason I like to use it is its novel quality. While I'm not there to entertain my clients, I acknowledge a contributing factor to any programme's success is adherence and application. So if we can make the session more fun while remaining effective, that's great.

LOADING

I don't like to use too many reps because the movement quality will drop. If you get a big drop in power you're losing the effectiveness of the exercise. If I'm using it early in a workout I'll do 3-5 sets of 3-5 reps with full rest between sets because it's not about testing fitness or the ability to recover. It's about generating force. The total amount of volume I'd do in a single session when training for power is in the region of 20 reps.

If I'm using it later in the workout then I might do three sets of 10 reps. In that instance the power will drop somewhat but it's still a valid exercise and it will get the heart rate up.

Overhead scoop throw

This is my personal favourite for developing explosive power – even more so than the Olympic lifts. The reason is that it involves uninhibited triple extension. When you do an Olympic lift you have to catch the bar, which involves controlling the bar and decelerating to complete the move. With this and all types of throw, you don't have to control the deceleration. It's also incredibly easy to teach and learn. I could teach 20 people to do this move in less than one session. The only catch is that you're going to need a lot of space.

I reserve this exercise for athletes and individuals who want to increase their rate of force development and become more explosive. It's a bit more awkward to set up and carry out than slams and it is slightly more complex so it needs to be used a bit more judiciously. It works well because you can quantify how well you're doing by seeing how far the ball has been thrown. That also makes it a good one to use if you have a group of competitive people because you can try to beat each other.

It's a move that I find everyone enjoys doing and it tends to have a positive impact on the application and attitude within a session. I reserve this move for after you've warmed up as a primer for the main lift of the session and as a CNS activator. I do not use it in metabolic conditioning circuits.

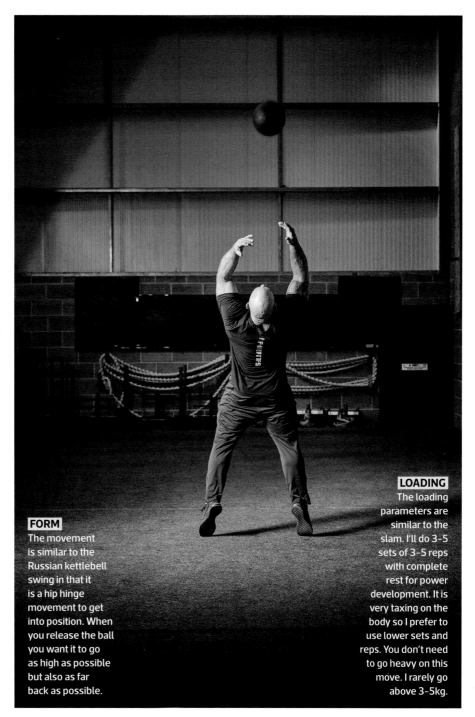

FORM
The movement is similar to the Russian kettlebell swing in that it is a hip hinge movement to get into position. When you release the ball you want it to go as high as possible but also as far back as possible.

LOADING
The loading parameters are similar to the slam. I'll do 3-5 sets of 3-5 reps with complete rest for power development. It is very taxing on the body so I prefer to use lower sets and reps. You don't need to go heavy on this move. I rarely go above 3-5kg.

Prowlers and sleds

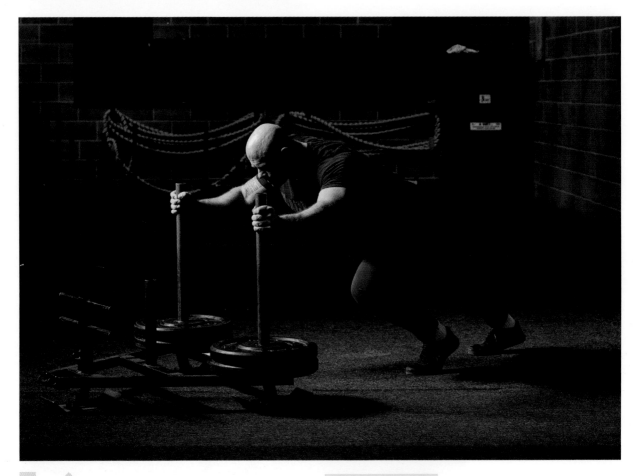

Sprinting is perhaps the ultimate way to generate power. It's the highest velocity that the human body can move so it is a tremendous stimulus. It's a whole-body exercise that recruits fast-twitch muscle fibres and can also burn fat – but most clients I see aren't track-ready and are likely to pull a hamstring if they burst into a full sprint. Using a prowler or sled for resisted sprints yields many of the benefits of sprinting, but with less chance of injury.

These moves are easy to learn and much less severe on the body. In my career I'm happy to admit that I've made many mistakes but I've never injured a client on a 10m prowler push or sled sprint. You can do them loaded or unloaded, but either way I prefer to do them over short distances in a powerful and aggressive way. If you do set after set then you'll eventually slow down and move into conditioning territory. If you're training for power you should recover fully between sets.

PROWLER PUSH

Adopt an athletic stance. Your shoulders should be higher than your hips and your body should be at about a 45° angle. If your hands are too low you'll put your force into the floor and the prowler won't move as efficiently or as quickly. Grip the frame as tightly as possible to create tension throughout the body so it's transferred through the torso, arms and into the prowler. Your knees should drive straight up and down to create forward momentum. I don't want to see any lateral movement. If your stride length is too long you'll get fatigued but if it's too short you won't generate enough force.

To develop power you want a short distance – maybe 10m. I want you to cover the distance as explosively and as violently as possible. The quality of the set is determined by how quickly you move. I also want you to explode into action, rather than building up speed. That's one of the reasons you

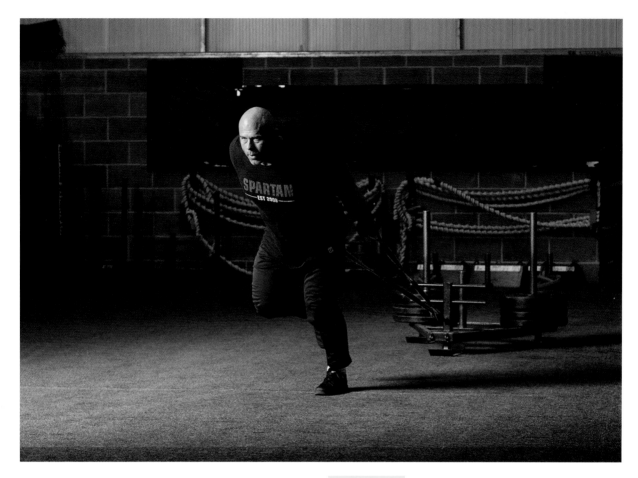

SLED PULL

should only do this after you have completed a full-body warm-up. If you're able to, set up prowler races because it's a great way to bring out people's competitive instincts.

LOADING PARAMETERS
Do **6–10** sets of **10m**

As always I'm looking for quality over quantity so I want full recovery between sets. If it takes 3 seconds to do the first set and 6 seconds to do the third, your power has dropped. I like to track sprint times and subsequent drop-off so I can programme individuals accordingly. I'd start with an empty prowler but you can add load as you progress. Just be careful not to allow the load on the sled to negatively impact form or speed – the maximum time you should work per set is 6 seconds.

As with the prowler push, adopt an athletic stance, leaning forwards as if you were about to do a standing start for a sprint. Start with small strides and build your stride length as you progress. If you overstrike you'll tend to move laterally and lose forward momentum. One cue I give people is to imagine that the floor is a giant treadmill that isn't switched on so they have to generate the force to move the belt themselves by driving hard into the floor and pushing it away. Throughout the pull your arms should be straight and directly behind your body.

LOADING PARAMETERS
Do **4–10** sets of **10m**

The same principles apply to the sled drag as they do to the prowler push. Aim for a maximum 6 seconds per set.

Weightlifting for strength training

Once someone has a solid strength foundation their training becomes increasingly focused on slow muscle contractions in moves such as squats, deadlifts and bench presses. What I want to do is keep progressing them and keep pushing them on, and that's why I introduce power training.

Earlier in this chapter we used power moves to excite the central nervous system and increase rate of force development. The jumps, throws and sprints discussed are all highly effective at doing so. Now is when I consider incorporating variations of the Olympic lifts to further develop power. Note I said 'consider' and 'variations'. The Olympic lifts are awesome for power development IF PERFORMED WITH COMPETENT TECHNIQUE! The vast majority of the strength training population simply can't perform them to this level, which includes many CrossFit enthusiasts I encounter.

Olympic lifting is a sport in itself. If you want to compete in that sport then I'll coach you in those lifts and I'll coach you in a completely different way to my general strength training clients, some of whom I only see once a week. Believe me, teaching them how to snatch really is not the best use of their time if their overall goal is to lose fat and add a bit of muscle.

Just because the Olympic lifts yield great results for competitive weightlifters doesn't mean they are automatically the best choice for all of my clients. You'd end up spending too much time on technique for the sessions to be productive and there would be very little stimulus through progressive overload. You have to do a needs analysis. What does the individual client need? If I'm trying to get someone stronger then I'll get them proficient in the foundation lifts, choose applicable barbell lifts and then select the assistance accordingly.

Some coaches like to include a bit of everything in their sessions so they'll have their clients attempt the full Olympic lifts. In my experience, when you do that, technique is often severely lacking and if that's the case then progress is going to be minimal and injuries highly likely. In my opinion, if you're getting a client to try to power clean two sessions in, you're not focusing on them or what they need to do to achieve their goals – you're trying to show off.

If you go too early with these lifts, what happens is that you end up pulling with improper technique. You're not pulling properly from the floor so there's minimal strength gains. But most importantly you're not catching the bar in the right position. So what happens? Normally you end up with an unimpressive power clean and sore wrists, elbows and shoulders. You become a physiotherapist's dream. That makes no sense to me. I love flipping 500kg tyres but that doesn't mean I fit it into every single programme that I create. Don't get me wrong, I love the Olympic lifts and I love watching them being performed well. But just because something looks badass doesn't mean everyone has to include it in their programme.

FEEL THE FORCE

I have not included the snatch and the clean and jerk in this section. If we're thinking about all-round strength training, the aim isn't to make someone a better weightlifter. I do, however, see value in everyone learning some key variations such as lifts from hang or pulls from blocks because the bang for your buck is higher. The number one goal for me with these movements is to increase the rate of force development, getting the person more powerful and explosive. That, in turn, will facilitate an increase in strength, which is always the priority.

This section focuses on the weightlifting variations that will have the biggest impact on your progress because they are efficient and produce a great training stimulus with a reduced chance of injury. Just because they aren't the full snatch or clean and jerk doesn't mean they're easy. Sure, they are simpler than the full lift, but never confuse simple with easy. They're all highly technical lifts and, like every other exercise in this book, they demand maximum focus and application.

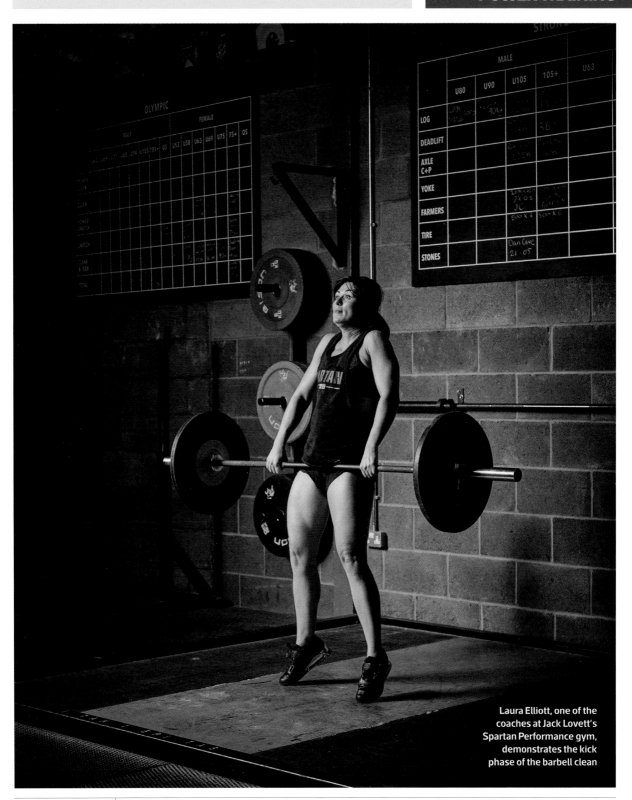

Laura Elliott, one of the coaches at Jack Lovett's Spartan Performance gym, demonstrates the kick phase of the barbell clean

Power snatch from hang

The key objective with this move is to commit to an explosive
hip drive and to move as fast as possible. You're also looking to
generate force using the posterior chain, something that's often
neglected because you can't see those muscles in the mirror. A
strong posterior chain has a tremendous crossover to other areas of
your training. If you increase your lower back, glute and hamstring
strength then your squat and deadlift will go up. In fact, pretty much
every exercise in this book would benefit from a stronger posterior
chain. And I'm willing to bet that every reader of this book would
also benefit from having a stronger posterior chain.

Unless you're an elite strength athlete, the main difference
between the clean and the snatch from hang is the hand position.
The hand position for the snatch grip is much wider and that will
place an extra emphasis on your grip strength which, as we've
already seen, will have a positive effect on your other lifts because
grip is often the weak link in the strength chain. The snatch-grip
version also increases upper back recruitment so that's useful if
you're trying to develop that muscle group.

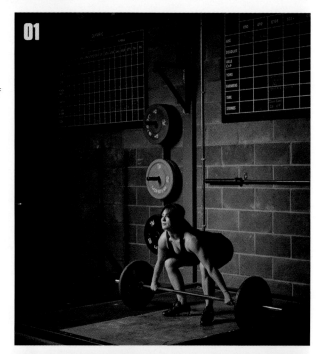

PERFECT FORM

- Set up with your shins close and the barbell over the mid-foot.
  Your feet should be about hip-width apart. Brace your core
  while standing, then perform a Romanian deadlift (RDL) or
  hinge to the knees, and finish the descent by squatting to the
  bar and gripping with hands wider than shoulder width in a
  snatch-width grip. A hook grip is optional but recommended.
- Your eyes should be looking forward and your neck straight
  in a neutral spine position. Brace again, ensuring your
  lats are locked down to stiffen the core even further, with
  grip tight and arms straight. Stand up with the barbell,
  keeping it as close to your body as possible. Your glutes
  should be squeezed from the outset and especially
  as the bar travels past your knees to lock-out.
- Hinge at the hips to send the bar down the front of your
  thighs until you feel a strong stretch in your hamstrings.
  Keep your shoulders back and use your lats to prevent
  the bar from losing touch with your thighs.
- Start to straighten back up and, as the bar reaches the
  top of your thighs, use hip drive to give momentum
  to its upward path. Make sure you go into triple
  extension of the hips, knees and ankles.
- Use a shrugging movement to aid the movement of the bar
  while bending at the elbows to keep the bar close to your body.
- As the bar starts to decelerate, drop under it while punching
  the load overhead and catch it in a quarter squat with
  your arms straight while trying to spread the bar. Once
  you have stabilised the weight, drive hard out of this
  position to stand up straight with the bar overhead.

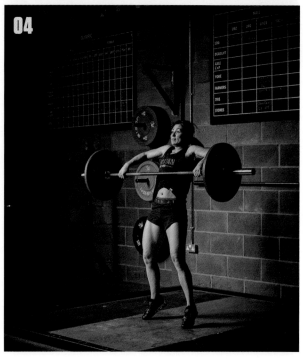

COACHING INSIGHT Some people simply find it easier to perform a power snatch than they do a power clean. I often find that's the case when I'm training strongmen. They are used to pulling with their arms, so when they perform a clean the arms have a tendency to take over. That's not really possible with the snatch grip because your arms are pretty much forced to be straight.

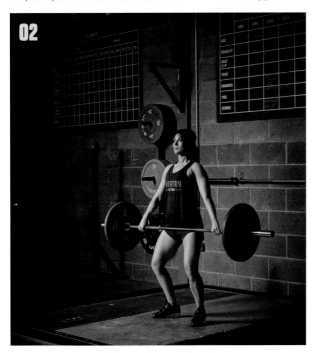

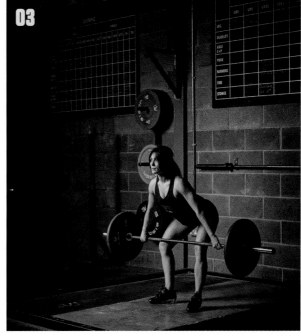

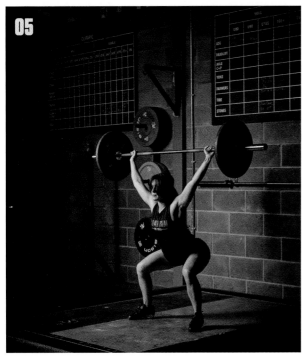

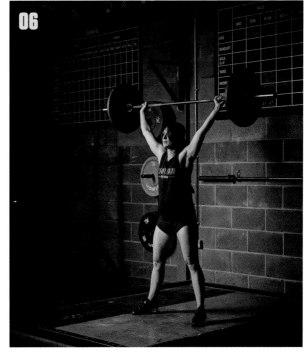

Power clean from hang

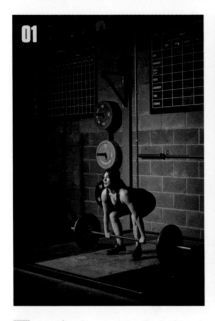

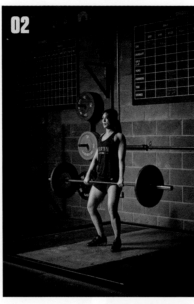

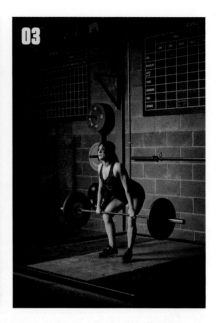

I want anyone doing Olympic lifts to perform them as aggressively as possible. I want you to really explode into triple extension. Once again, this is very much about how you move the weight, rather than focusing on your one-rep max. Technique and speed should always trump weight on the bar. There's more value in a fast, technically sound clean than a reverse-curl-to-front-squat-good morning performed badly but with slightly more weight. So be prudent in terms of how you load – most Olympic lifts can be considered strength-speed movements, performed with moderate to heavy weights.

A lot of people struggle with wrist flexibility to hold the bar in the rack position, especially if they have come to weightlifting later in their training life. My advice would be to work all aspects of wrist and forearm mobility, including the four drills shown here.

PERFECT FORM

- Stand with your shins close and the barbell over the mid-foot. Your feet should be about hip width apart. Brace your core while standing, then perform an RDL or hinge to the knees, and finish the descent by squatting to the bar and gripping with hands shoulder-width apart or slightly wider with an overhand grip. A hook grip is optional but recommended.
- Your eyes should be looking forwards and your neck straight in a neutral spine position. Brace again, ensuring your the lats are locked down to stiffen the core even further, with grip tight and arms straight. Stand up with the barbell, keeping it as close to your body as possible. Your glutes should be squeezed from the outset and especially as the bar travels past the knees to lock-out.
- Hinge at the hips to send the bar down the front of your thighs until you feel a strong stretch in your hamstrings. Keep your shoulders back and use your lats to prevent the bar from losing touch with your thighs.
- Start to straighten back up and, as the bar reaches the top of your thighs, use hip drive to give momentum to its upward path. Make sure you go into triple extension of the hips, knees and ankles.
- Use a shrugging movement to aid the movement of the bar while punching your elbows up and dropping under the bar to catch it high on the shoulders and not the wrists.
- Keeping your elbows high and with an upright torso, drive hard out of this position to return to standing.

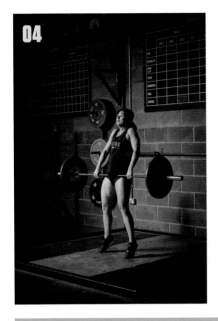
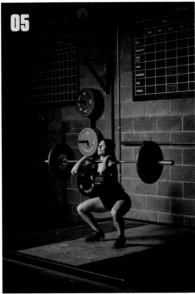
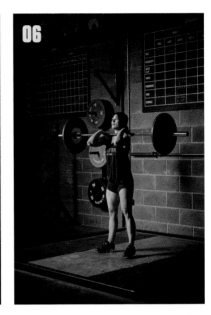

MOBILITY DRILLS

Practise these drills, starting with stage 1 and progressing to stage 4 if you struggle to get into the rack position. They're highly effective drills but very demanding for the uninitiated.

Progress from 1 to 4 at your own pace. Always be careful to not stretch too hard and injure yourself. Regardless of the benefits, such positions can be unforgiving if used incorrectly.

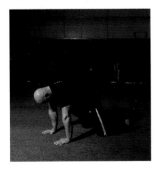
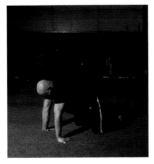
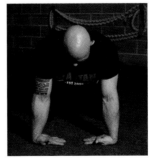
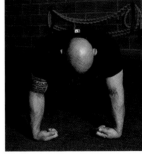

STAGE 1
Keep your elbows locked, palms flat and fingers forwards. Before a workout, rock back and forth on your hips dynamically. Hold each end range for post-workout static stretches.

STAGE 2
Keep your elbows locked, palms flat and fingers backwards. Before a workout, rock back and forth on your hips dynamically. Hold each end range for post-workout static stretches.

STAGE 3
Keeping your elbows locked, place the backs of your hands on the floor just inside shoulder width, with your fingers facing towards each other. Hold that position as a stretch.

STAGE 4
From the position described previously, make fists with both hands. Hold these fists for a few seconds then release and repeat.

Snatch and clean variations from blocks

I like to get people lifting from the hang before they lift from blocks. Lifts from the hang are slightly more technical, though less technical than those from the floor. They also have the added benefit of an eccentric phase (lowering the bar to the starting position) and a transition from eccentric to concentric. This eccentric action as you lower into the hang provides a

pre-stretch which can increase force production. When you pull from blocks, you're pulling a dead weight every rep. You must go from zero muscle activity to maximum power output instantly. This a great way to develop starting strength.

When you lift from blocks you will probably be able to lift heavier weights than you can from hang. And because this is just

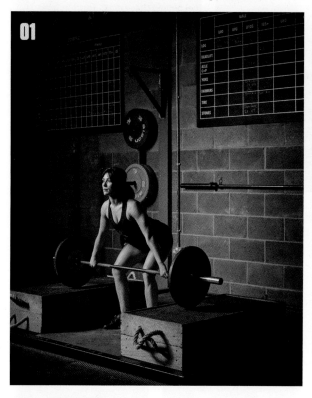

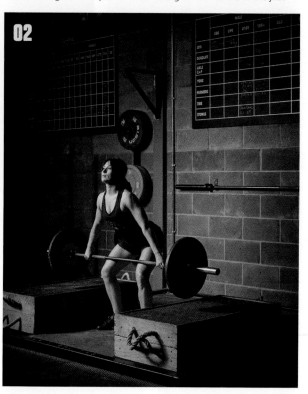

PERFECT FORM SNATCH PULL FROM BLOCKS

- Set the blocks so that the bar is just above or just below knee height when you're in the start position. To get into the start position, stand with your shins close and the barbell over the mid-foot. Your feet should be about hip-width apart.
- Brace your core while standing, then perform an RDL or hinge to the bar, gripping with hands wider than shoulder width in a snatch-width grip. A hook grip is optional but recommended.
- Your eyes should be looking forwards and your neck straight in a neutral spine position. Brace again, ensuring your lats are locked down to stiffen the core even further, with grip tight and arms straight.

- With tension on the bar and your core braced, lift the bar off the blocks. Start to straighten up and, as the bar reaches the top of your thighs, use hip drive to give momentum to its upward path. Make sure you go into triple extension of the hips, knees and ankles.
- Use a shrugging movement to aid the movement of the bar while bending at the elbows to keep the bar as close to your body as possible.

a pull with no deceleration into a catch position required, you can really go into uninhibited triple extension. That's why this lift is great for people who aren't necessarily good at weightlifting but would benefit from increased posterior chain development. Snatch pulls from blocks are a personal favourite for my own training and a lot of the strongman and strongwoman athletes I work with.

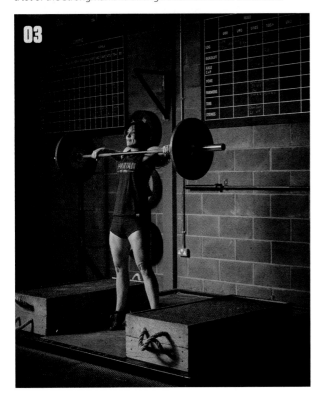

BLOCKS CHALLENGES

CHASING WEIGHT
Pulls from blocks are less technical than those from the hang so you tend to encounter fewer issues. What I do find is that people chase weight and, as a result, don't go into proper triple extension. They start to pull with their arms to compensate and when that happens they're not getting the full benefit of the exercise. The arms should be like rope – merely connecting you to the bar. I don't want to see the move turn into a reverse curl.

PULLING TOO HIGH
The other issue I see is people pulling too high. The highest the bar should be is level with the clavicle. It's fine to pull to the sternum if you're going into triple extension. It's a bit like a kettlebell swing in that respect –you're not chasing height. I judge the quality of the exercise by whether the glutes are contracted.

POOR START POSITION
If your start position isn't optimal and you're not properly over the bar, you're fighting a losing battle. If you're too far behind the bar it'll put your weight on your heels and when that happens it's a lot harder to get into triple extension.

PERFECT FORM POWER CLEAN FROM BLOCKS

- Set the blocks so that the bar is either just below or just above knee height when you're in the start position. To get into the start position, stand with your shins close and the barbell over the mid-foot. Your feet should be about hip-width apart.
- Brace your core while standing, then perform an RDL or hinge to the bar, gripping with hands shoulder-width apart or slightly wider with an overhand grip. A hook grip is optional but recommended.
- Your eyes should be looking forwards and your neck straight in a neutral spine position. Brace again, ensuring your lats are locked down to stiffen the core even further, with grip tight and arms straight.

- With tension on the bar and your core braced, lift the bar off the blocks. Start to straighten up and, as the bar reaches the top of your thighs,use hip drive to give momentum to its upward path. Make sure you go into triple extension of the hips, knees and ankles.
- Use a shrugging movement to aid the movement of the bar while bending at the elbows to keep the bar close to your body.
- Aim to get the bar as high as possible, up to chin height. If it is going higher than that, that's a sign that you're ready for a heavier load.
- Control the descent of the bar to 'catch' it in your hips and reset fully before performing the next rep.

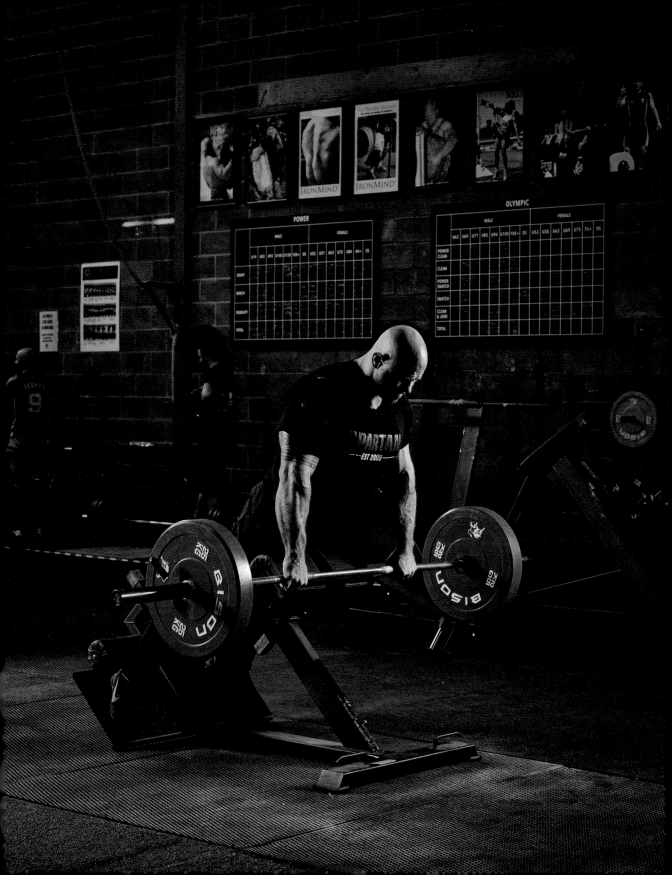

05.

↙

HYPERTROPHY EXERCISES

Strength and hypertrophy go hand in hand. They complement each other perfectly. I'm an advocate of the saying, 'a stronger muscle has a greater potential to be a bigger muscle' – and vice versa, assuming you train both of those qualities effectively. You cannot optimise one quality without the other.

Heavy barbell lifts are an excellent way of building maximal strength but that can be enhanced by a judicious selection of accessory lifts for hypertrophy. Hypertrophy movements act to build the muscles, whereas the main lifts in this book focus on the capacity to use said muscles.

Building as much muscle as possible is a desirable objective because it's almost like armour. I want someone who not just performs but who also looks like they can perform too. That's the holy grail. Everyone wants to look better naked and there's nothing wrong with that. What I don't advocate is if that comes at the cost of strength being sacrificed. But, if you train smart, I don't see why that should happen.

ZERO IN ON WEAKNESS

Hypertrophy methods can also help to strengthen weaknesses identified in the main barbell lifts. Maybe you're weak at lock-out on the bench press, or maybe you struggle breaking the floor in the deadlift. Hypertrophy lifts, when selected and performed intelligently, can develop those weak areas and bring balance to the body; that's not only good for aesthetics, it will also sustain longer-term gains on the strength lifts while minimising the risk of injury. Even if your goals are purely strength-based, you cannot pursue your goals if you're injured – and that injury may not be down to a technique flaw but a muscular imbalance.

We can induce a certain amount of hypertrophy with the foundation moves alone and that's where we start. Getting stronger in the key barbell exercises will also build muscle. I like proven methods and as a result, I'm a strong believer in the basics when it comes to building muscle. That's why most of the hypertrophy moves in this section involve a barbell, dumbbell or your bodyweight. All too often when it comes to training for strength or hypertrophy people are looking for the next best thing but they are usually looking at the icing on the cake. You can't concern yourself with that until you have maximised the return from the basics.

Once you have exploited the benefits of the basic barbell lifts for hypertrophy, you can explore the supplementary lifts. Even then, it takes a long time to exhaust the potential of a machine, a cable or a dumbbell just on sets of 10 reps with varying tempo, and that's what you need to do before you start to concern yourself with the benefits of things such as bench press with hanging band technique. That technique is for specific people at a specific stage.

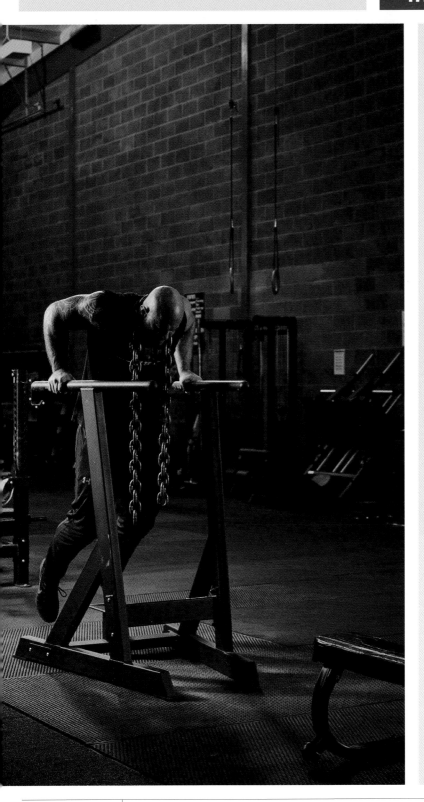

Takeaway tips

FOCUS ON TEMPO

How you execute each rep is key for stimulating hypertrophy. We're trying to create muscle damage so a controlled, even slow, eccentric (lowering) phase is essential. I also want you to control the concentric (lifting) phase. You're not using the same technique that you used in the power training or even the key lifts section. As always, I'm not particularly interested in the number of sets and reps you perform. I'm more interested in how you perform each rep. I pay attention to how bodybuilders perform their reps and the good ones never sacrifice quality while chasing rep count. Remember – your muscles can't count reps. They respond to the tension that's placed on them.

GET A MIND-MUSCLE CONNECTION

I want you to use the exercises in this section to really feel the target muscle. You're not simply moving weight from A to B. You want to really feel the target muscle working. This is where maturity and training experience comes into play and it is vital to get good habits ingrained at the start. If you look at the bodybuilder and coach John Meadows, he does many exercises that most people do, but it is how he does them that counts. He milks every last gram of benefit from every single rep.

LEAVE YOUR EGO AT THE DOOR

This means I'd rather you used 40kg on the bent-over row and did it perfectly than you used 100kg and did some bastardised version. But that's not a licence to permanently lift too light. I don't want you to be a pussy. To make a muscle grow you don't just walk into the gym and it magically happens. It's how you commit to the reps that counts. The body doesn't want to change, it likes homeostasis, so you've got to put it under sufficient stress. Building muscle is a tough ask so you need to commit fully to the process.

Squat assistance

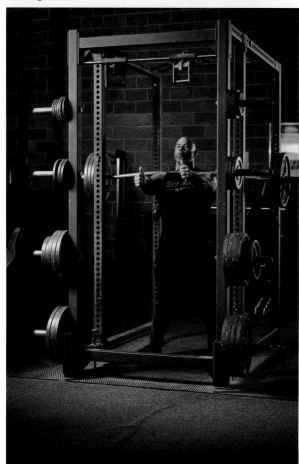
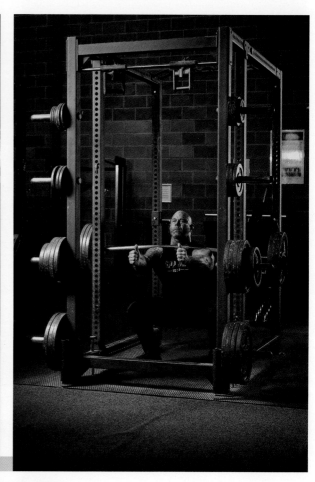

FRANKENSTEIN SQUAT

This is my personal favourite squat variation. It's similar to the front squat, but it requires an even greater focus on form, bar placement and torso rigidity. There truly can't be any weak links from head to toe when performing a rep.

This variation encourages the use of a pause at the bottom of the lift. And when I say pause, I'm not talking about a split second – I'm talking between 3 and 9 seconds. I'd recommend starting with a 3-second pause and then adding two more seconds every week until you get to a 9-second pause. The pause is really good for teaching people to execute and maintain a core brace. You also get an extra upper back stimulus. The pause will limit the load but that means it allows you to get a useful training effect while using a lighter load.

PERFECT FORM

- Take the bar out of the rack, resting it on the front of your shoulders with your arms straight out in front of you, thumbs pointing up. Position your feet just outside shoulder width, with your toes turned slightly out.
- Brace your core, screwing your feet into the floor as if trying to spread the floor.
- Initiate the squat by driving your knees out and forwards slightly, lowering into the bottom position. Here, you should be stable and pause briefly, with hips below the knees and back tight.
- Return to standing, making sure to drive your knees out and screwing your feet into the ground.

EXPERT TIP
Sometimes you want to load up the bar with as much weight as possible but at other times it's useful to get a training response with a lighter load because it places less of a demand on your CNS.

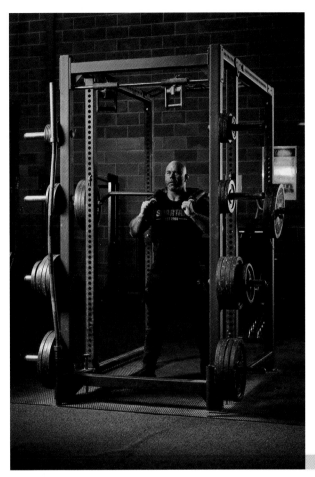
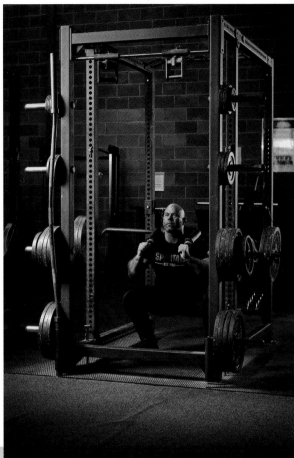

SAFETY BAR SQUAT

This is a valuable variation for anyone who has had an upper arm or shoulder injury that rules out straight-bar squatting. You retain all the benefits of a straight-bar squat and since the bar wants to tip you forwards, the torso musculature and stabilisers have to work even harder to keep you in a good position.

PERFECT FORM

- Stand tall with the safety bar across the top of your traps, holding it by the handles with your elbows pointing forwards and your upper arms parallel to the floor. Position your feet just outside shoulder width, with your toes turned slightly out.
- Brace your core, screwing your feet into the floor as if trying to spread the floor.
- Initiate the squat by driving your knees out and pulling your hamstrings back to lower into the bottom position. Here, you should be stable and pause briefly, with hips below the knees and back tight.
- Return to standing, making sure to drive your knees out and pulling your elbows back and down, keeping your torso as rigid as possible.

EXPERT TIP

Grip the handles tightly. Despite the comfort of the pad, you do not want to lose your upper back tension. While important on the descent this is even more so as you squat back up. Do not allow the bar to tip you forwards.

Squat assistance

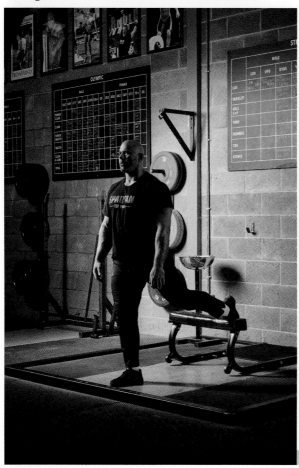

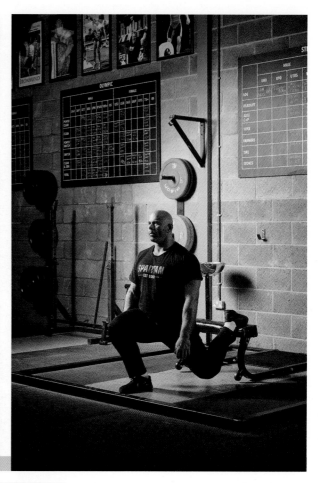

BULGARIAN SPLIT SQUAT

Now, I accept that this isn't most people's favourite exercise because it is awkward to balance and burns like hell, but it offers some excellent training benefits. For hypertrophy, I'm fond of a slow eccentric – maybe 3-6 seconds per rep. If you want more quad emphasis the knee on your lead leg can go over the ankle, as long as the front foot stays flat on the floor. And if you want more glute and hamstring development, set up so that the lead foot is below your knee and your shin is vertical. I recommend placing a soft pad under your knee that comes down to the floor – but make sure that you don't bounce off it.

PERFECT FORM

- Place one foot on a bench behind you with your other foot slightly in front of you. Add load if required with a dumbbell or kettlebell in each hand.
- Squat down through the front leg, keeping your foot flat on the ground and your rear leg bent. Ensure that your knee does not crash into the floor.
- Drive up evenly through your front foot, ensuring it remains flat on the floor at all times. Do not tip forwards onto your toes.

EXPERT TIP

I like my clients to perform this exercise barefoot to take advantage of the ankle mobility and stability effects. It's a hard exercise to balance so that makes it great for developing proprioception too.

EXPERT TIP I frequently use the unilateral leg press because most people have strength imbalances and this is a good way to address them. It really helps if you have a machine that has independent plates so you can work one leg at a time.

LEG PRESS

PERFECT FORM

- Adjust the machine so when seated you're positioned correctly and safely. Position your feet against the platform with your feet hip-width apart, your toes pointing slightly outwards and your legs straight.
- Unhook the safety catch or catches, grip the handles hard, then bend your knees to lower them towards your torso. Allow your knees to come slightly to the side of your torso, not straight down.
- Once in the bottom position push through your heels to straighten your legs and return to the top position. Never lock out the knees at the top. Keep them slightly bent with tension on the leg musculature itself.

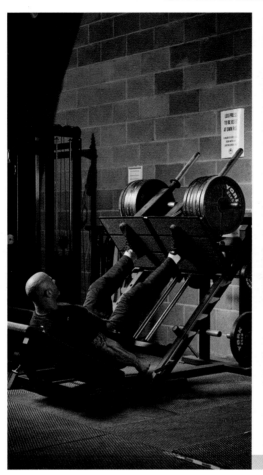
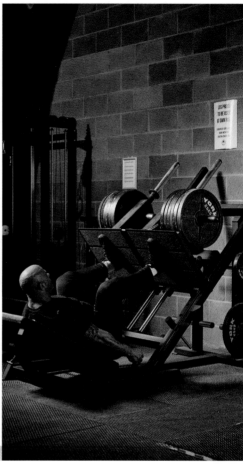

My first rule with a leg press is to avoid locking out your knees. If you want to know why, just go on YouTube and search for leg press fails! Having a slight bend in the knees will also keep the tension on your muscles, which is the point of the exercise.

I also see many people lower the weight too far – remember this isn't a flexibility test. You don't want your lower back to round and come off the pad. If I can fit my hand between your lower back and the pad, that's a sign that you've lost control of your lumbar spine.

How you place your feet will determine the training effect of the exercise. When your feet are close together that will emphasise your VMO. When the feet are wide it targets the outside of the quads and when they are shoulder width you get a more even development. That is, of course, a generalisation but it's a useful one. I recommend experimenting with different foot positions and I also encourage clients to adjust their foot position within sets. I might get someone to do 12 reps narrow, 12 reps shoulder width and 12 reps wide in the same set. You can vary the height of the foot placement too. The higher your feet, the more you emphasise your glutes and hamstrings. The further down you go, the more you hit your quads.

This knowledge will help you use the exercise more wisely so that, for example, on deadlift day, you could perform a leg press with your feet high to target your glutes and hamstrings. Then on a squat day you place them lower to target the quads.

Overhead press assistance

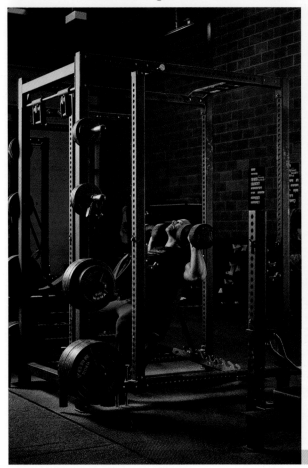
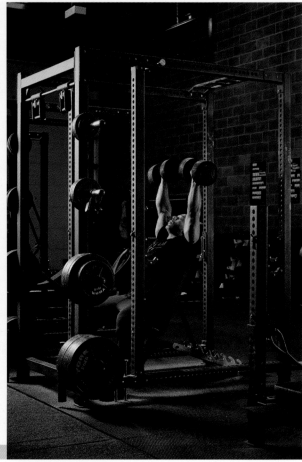

SEATED DUMBBELL PRESS

Doing this exercise with your back supported and a solid foot position means that you can overload your delts and triceps in a big way. Dumbbells allow a freedom of movement that a barbell can't give you. You don't have to use a pronated grip, where your palms are facing forwards; my preference is for a neutral, semi-supinated grip where your wrists are at 45°. I find that grip is kinder on the shoulder joints and also allows you to overload the triceps, which is crucial for pressing strength. But essentially you'll have to find the right grip for your biomechanics and your training aims.

Another benefit of using dumbbells is that your hands aren't fixed at a certain width apart as they are with a barbell. You can bring them together above your head to maximise the effectiveness of the muscle contraction – but don't smash the weights together because that will take tension off the muscle. Aim to control the entire movement – a vital skill to learn if hypertrophy is your goal.

PERFECT FORM

- Sit on a bench set in the upright position and hold a pair of dumbbells by your shoulders, using a neutral grip.
- Brace your core and press the weights directly overhead, taking care to ensure that they don't bang into each other at the top of the move.
- Lower the weights back to the start under control.

EXPERT TIP

I prefer to see your palms facing in at the start. With experience you can start to exploit the versatility that dumbbells offer. What's comfortable for you will depend on the individual – there are no hard and fast rules about what grip you should take.

LATERAL RAISE

The biggest favour you can do yourself is leaving your ego at the door when it comes to this lift. I see so many guys trying to lift a weight that's too heavy and end up just swinging it around. All that will do is ensure that you don't engage the muscle and give yourself shoulder issues. I can't stress this enough – it's not about what you lift it's about how you lift it. I want you to feel the muscle working, so use a slow and controlled movement and think about time under tension.

- Stand holding a dumbbell in each hand on the outside of your thighs.
- Initiating the movement using your middle delts, raise both arms up to your sides, leading with the little finger on each hand.
- Raise the dumbbells to shoulder height, then lower them under control, rather than letting gravity take over.

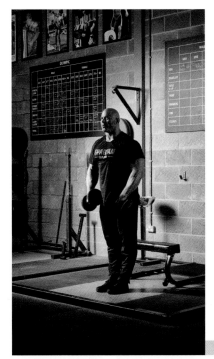
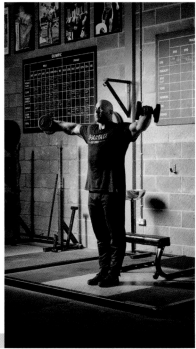

FRONT RAISE

This is similar to the lateral raise in how you should approach and execute it, and it's an excellent tool for anterior delt development which ultimately leads to bigger overhead presses. This has been a very effective exercise for me over the years and certainly facilitates a strong press.

- Stand holding a dumbbell in each hand on the front of your thighs.
- Alternate raising each arm in front of you with the backs of your hands facing the ceiling.
- Raise the dumbbell to shoulder height or just above, then lower under control. Alternate arms with each rep.

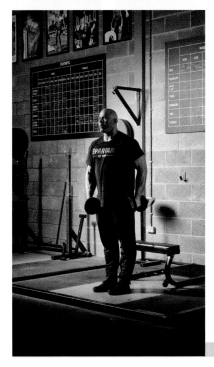
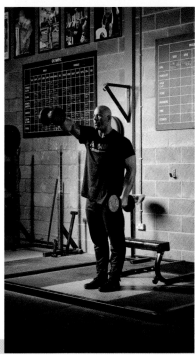

Overhead press assistance

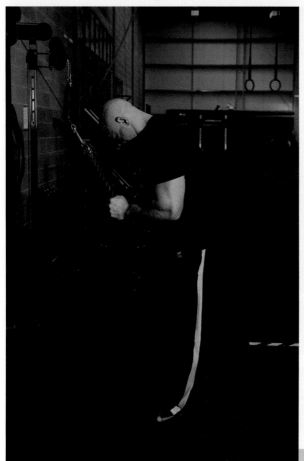 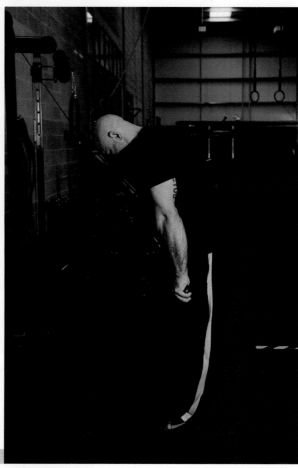

CABLE TRICEPS PRESS-DOWN

Whenever you're doing a cable move try to use the cable as an interactive coaching tool. If you're moving erratically, the cable will oscillate and not feel smooth and that means that the tension on the muscle isn't consistent. Don't go for the heaviest weight you think you can lift – go lighter and focus on controlling the movement. Your aim is to exert continuous tension on the target muscle. It's also important to not let gravity take over when you're lowering the weight stack and miss out on the benefits of the eccentric portion of the lift.

PERFECT FORM

- Position the cable high on the machine and use a rope attachment.
- Get into the start position with your body upright, your core braced, your elbows tight to your sides and your forearms at right angles to your upper arms.
- Ensure that there is tension in the cable before you start then, with minimal upper arm movement, straighten your arms before pulling the rope apart at the bottom of the move to maximise the triceps contraction.
- Return to the start, controlling the movement throughout and keeping your elbows tight to your sides for the duration of the exercise.

EXPERT TIP
I want sustained tension on the triceps, using a 3-second concentric and eccentric. Mind-muscle connection is important – really feel the triceps contraction, otherwise the chest and front shoulder can easily become dominant.

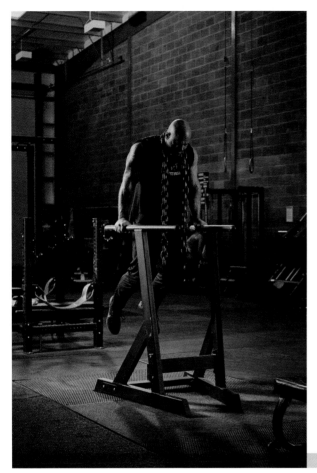
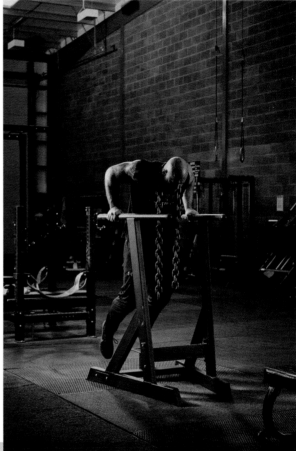

TRICEPS DIP

I like to perform these using fat bars because the thicker the bar, the more comfortable they are to hold. Just make sure that you don't move like a jackhammer or a woodpecker. We want smooth, good-quality reps. You can also add extra load by using a dip belt or chains around your neck. I find both of those options are more comfortable than a dumbbell between your feet.

The dip is sometimes referred to as the upper body squat and I kind of buy into that, but it isn't necessarily appropriate for everyone. Some people don't have the shoulder health to perform them correctly so you need to judge if it is worth doing the exercise. In short, if it causes pain, find an alternative move.

PERFECT FORM

- Grip the parallel bars.
- Bend at the elbows and lower under control, keeping them tight to your sides and avoiding them flaring out, until they are at an angle greater than 90°.
- Press back up smoothly to the start and repeat the exercise.

EXPERT TIP

I like to develop neck strength and having a chain around your neck and traps during dips will do just that. This move is particularly good for combat athletes and rugby players – and it looks cool.

Deadlift assistance

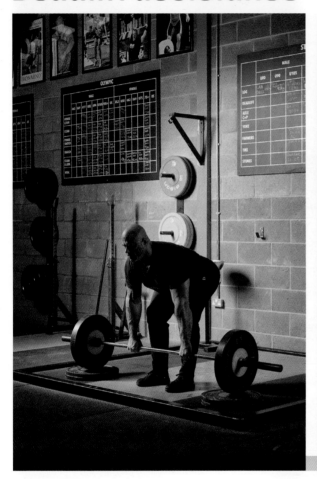
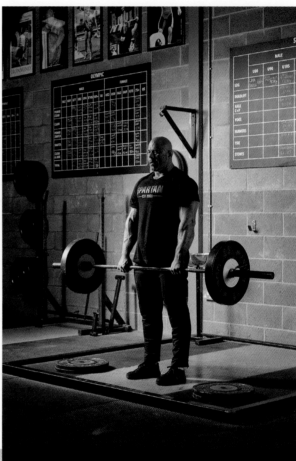

STIFF-LEGGED DEADLIFT

As with the Romanian deadlift, I want you take a double overhead grip. You can use straps because it's likely that this move will come at the end of a grip-intense session. If your grip is fatigued then you may find your ability to lift is compromised to the extent that you can't effectively challenge your hamstrings. If you're using it earlier in a session, try not to use straps.

Not everyone has the flexibility to get into the start position to lift off the floor so you may want to elevate the bar by, say, 10cm by placing it on blocks or weight plates. I like people to hinge into the start position and adjust from there.

PERFECT FORM

- Deadlift the bar into the start position, with hands just wider than shoulder width and the bar resting on the front of your thighs.
- Brace your core and, keeping the bar close to you, hinge at the hips to send the bar down the front of your thighs.
- Return to the floor with your legs almost straight but knees not locked, making sure you keep the weight in your heels and mid-foot and push your backside back to engage the hamstrings.
- Deadlift the bar back to standing position, keeping your legs straight, back tight and lats engaged and squeezing your glutes at the top of the rep.

EXPERT TIP
Use a double overhand grip and lift from a height from which you can get into a good position. This is because it's hard to maintain a tight back with stiff legs – it's all to make sure that you focus on form and technique.

EXPERT TIP Go only as low as you can go while maintaining a straight back and tension on the hamstrings. If this pulls on the back of your knees, consider a wider foot placement and turning you toes further out.

45 RAISE

I don't call this a back extension because it's more of a hip extension. I like to use a quad-supported hinge set-up because I want to emphasise the hamstrings and glutes. For loading weight, I prefer to use a barbell rather than a kettlebell or a dumbbell because it is easier to hold and easier to add load. I also find that it's not essential to go as low as you possibly can – instead, go as low as you can while maintaining a neutral spine.

- Position yourself so that you're angled at 45°, feet about shoulder-width apart and toes turned out.
- To lower, break at the hips, pushing them backwards while lowering your chest and keeping a straight lower back.
- Pull yourself back up to 45° by contracting the glutes hard, never losing torso rigidity in the process.

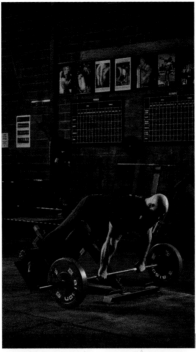
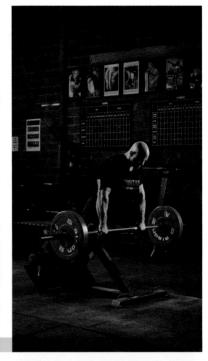

GLUTE/HAM RAISE

It's essential to master the eccentric portion of this lift first. So slow it down to a 5- to 6-second eccentric and just fight gravity. Build eccentric strength first and don't try to increase the load too soon. I often do three sets of ten reps just using bodyweight. You should also experiment with foot placement. Use narrow, medium and wide placements and also vary the toe angle. You might find that a certain foot position alleviates stress on the knees too.

- Position yourself in a glute/ham raise machine with your knees behind the pad and toes driven into the foot plate.
- Brace your core, contract your glutes and lower slowly under control.
- While staying in complete control of your movement, lower until your legs are straight, keeping the torso rigid. Return to upright by driving your toes into the foot plate and contracting your hamstrings, glutes and even your calves.

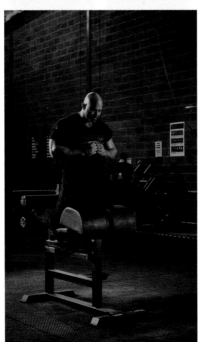
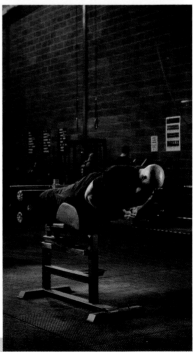

Bench press assistance

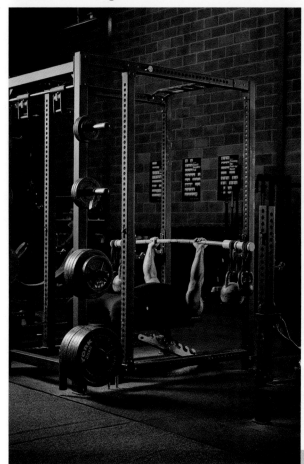
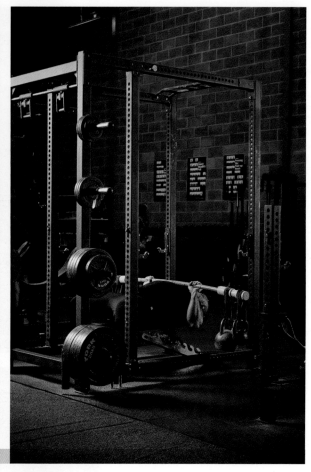

EARTHQUAKE BAR BENCH PRESS

An earthquake bar is a bar that reverberates when you move it. You can load it up by hanging a kettlebell, dumbbell or even a weight plate off each side using a band. The instability and the movement of the bar is excellent for your shoulder stability because the small muscles of your rotator cuff are constantly reacting to the change in stimulus. If you don't have access to an earthquake bar then you can achieve a similar effect with a conventional barbell but it isn't as good.

Make sure you start light. It isn't a pissing contest. I don't care how heavy you lift. I care about how well you control the bar. This isn't a move for beginners and there is no need to be competitive on this lift. It's all about the quality of the movement.

PERFECT FORM

- Set up on a flat bench with your feet planted slightly behind your knees (stance can be adjusted based on hip mobility and limb length), gripping the bar with an overhand grip, hands shoulder-width apart.
- With your chest up and your abs and glutes engaged, drive your feet into the floor and your head and shoulders into the bench to create full-body tension as you lower the bar towards your chest under control.
- Maintain this tension as you press the bar straight back up over your chest until your arms lock out.
- Aim to use a slow tempo and keep the bar path as smooth as possible, resisting the oscillation created by the bar. Use a vice-like grip at all times. Think 'white knuckles' as an effective coaching cue.

EXPERT TIP

Be humble, or the move will humble you. Start with relatively light weights, then add load gradually. I bench press about 230kg but I get mileage out of an earthquake bar using kettlebells of between 8 and 28kg each side.

EXPERT TIP This will develop core strength and stability, particularly if you are using heavy weights (50kg, say) because you use anti-rotational strength. The weight wants to pull your body off-balance so you have to resist that.

SINGLE-ARM BENCH PRESS

Everyone has a dominant side in the bench press so doing the one-arm version of the move will help to address that. You should train to strengthen the weaker side and aim to get to a point where you are able to perform the same number of reps with the same weight on both sides.

- Set up on a flat bench with your feet planted slightly behind your knees (stance can be adjusted based on individual hip mobility and limb length), gripping one dumbbell with a neutral grip and your arm straight.
- With your chest up and your abs and glutes engaged, drive your feet into the floor and your head and shoulders into the bench to create full-body tension as you lower the dumbbell towards the side of your chest under control.
- Maintain this tension as you press the dumbbell straight back up over your chest until your arms lock out. Make sure you resist the force pulling you out of alignment and don't let your torso rotate to one side. Having your opposite arm outstretched and rigid will help facilitate this.

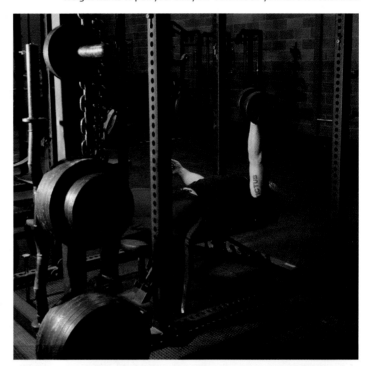

DUMBBELL BENCH PRESS

A neutral grip is my personal preference both for shoulder health and range of motion. While I like to progress the load lifted and not shy away from heavier sets, dumbbells are inherently tougher to stabilise than barbells and thus greater caution and control must be exhibited at all times. Be ambitious in your load selection, sure, but keep the ego in check. Rep quality always supersedes rep weight.

- Set up on a flat bench with your feet planted slightly behind your knees (stance can be adjusted based on individual hip mobility and limb length), gripping the dumbbells with a neutral grip with arms straight and hands shoulder-width apart.
- With your chest up and your abs and glutes engaged, drive your feet into the floor and your head and shoulders into the bench to create full-body tension as you lower the dumbbells towards the sides of your chest under control.
- Maintain this tension as you press the dumbbells straight back up over your chest until your arms lock out, taking care not to let the dumbbells clash at the top of the move.

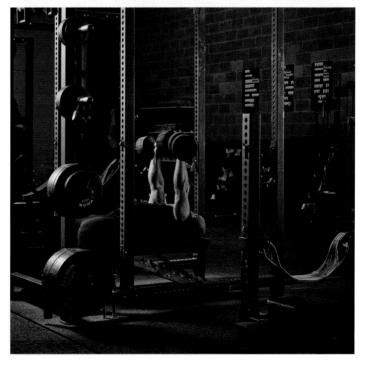

Back assistance

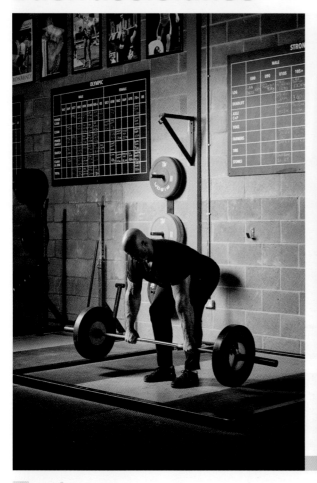

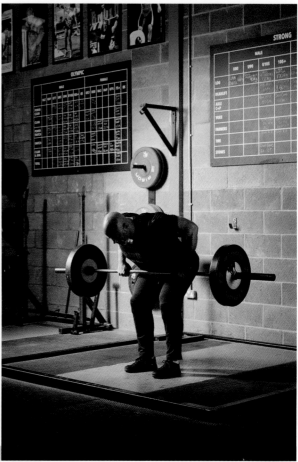

BENT-OVER ROW

This is my key assistance move for horizontal pulling. It requires significant torso strength, not just lats, and has a great carryover to deadlifting performance too. Just make sure it doesn't become an ugly RDL/upright row hybrid.

Again, while I advocate progressive overload, this can easily become an ego lift. I want a straight back and I don't want to see any torso movement. The prime mover is the arms – you're not pivoting at the hips.

A useful variation is the Pendlay row where the bar comes to a dead stop on the floor between reps. I consider that a progression because when the bar comes to a stop you have to move it with a more aggressive start than you do when using the stretch reflex component of a conventional bent-over row.

PERFECT FORM

- Grip a barbell in an overhand grip, with a similar width to that of your deadlift.
- With minimal torso movement, pull the bar to your stomach, keeping the elbows back and tight to the body.
- At the top of the movement, squeeze the upper back and lats while keeping the torso rigid and hip angle fixed. Aim to pull the bar into the body at this point, not just touching it.
- Lower the bar under control and repeat the exercise.

EXPERT TIP

This is easily one of the most bastardised moves I see. If I have 10 different people they'll perform 10 different versions. Focus on form – it requires discipline to lift light enough to ensure good form but heavy enough to elicit a training response.

EXPERT TIP I never advise people to use straps on this lift, regardless of where it comes in your workout. Not only does that reduce the likelihood of you lifting too heavy and thus sloppily, it also ensures that your grip strength is up to the task.

DUMBBELL BENT-OVER ROW

This is a great movement for both back and grip development. It is also easy to turn into an ego lift and I never want the pursuit of weight to compromise form. I prefer to see a controlled tempo with a two-second squeeze at the top of each rep. That gives you a great peak contraction but I rarely see anyone lift that way because they're only interested in the number on the dumbbell.

- Grip a dumbbell in an overhand grip, with your arm hanging straight from the shoulder. The opposite arm should be supported on a bench.
- With minimal torso movement, pull the dumbbell up to your sides, leading with your elbow and keeping it tight to your side.
- Squeeze your back muscles at the top of the move by trying to bring your shoulder blades together. Lower the weight under control.

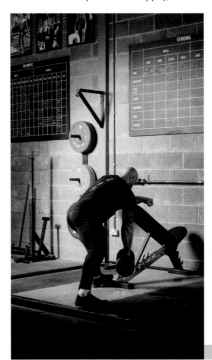
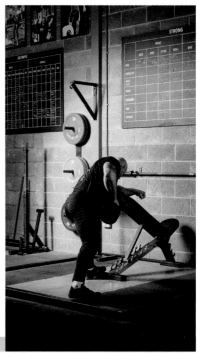

CHEST-SUPPORTED ROW

I like this move done using either a machine or a bench. There isn't much core engagement but it builds a big upper back and contracts the lats so it's a great way to overload the back musculature without taxing the lower back. I like the machine we have at Spartan Performance because you can adjust the handles. They rotate through 360° and that means you can, for example, start with a neutral grip and rotate your wrists as you lift the weight to maximise the quality of the muscle contraction.

- Let the bar hang down with straight arms, then row it up to your sides, leading with your elbows and keeping them tight to your sides.
- Squeeze your back muscles at the top of the move by trying to bring your shoulder blades together.
- Lower the weights under control.

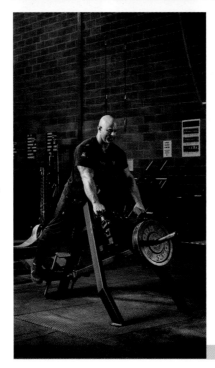
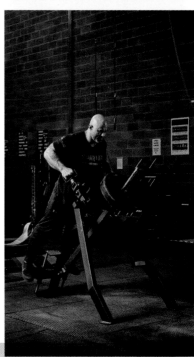

Back assistance

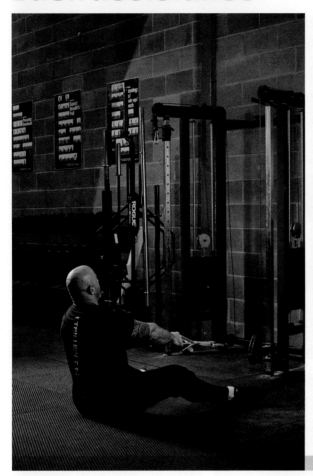
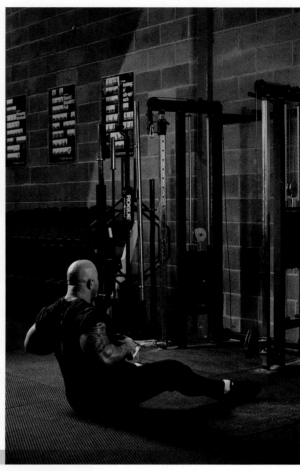

SEATED CABLE ROW

When used correctly, cables ensure a constant tension and thus stimulus on the targeted muscles at all times. Row and pull-down variations are an effective method to hit the back musculature from all angles, which is where barbells and dumbbells can fall short. You're aiming to target your lats here so don't use your legs or fall backwards to initiate the movement. I really like to do this move using an attachment called a MAG Grip because I find it really helps you to focus on contracting your lats.

PERFECT FORM

- Set the cable to a low height with a double grip and sit on the floor with your knees bent at 90° and your torso leaning back slightly.
- Start with your arms straight and tension in the cable, then brace your core and pull the cable towards your stomach, leading with your elbows and keeping your elbows tight to your sides. Pause at this point to maximise the muscular contraction.
- Keep your chest up throughout the pull and avoiding rocking your torso back to assist the movement.

EXPERT TIP

I want continuous tension through the cable. This move is to develop back thickness – I'm not trying to train your forearms so choose the grip that allows you to lift as much weight as possible. The angle of the MAG Grips' handles encourages more lat development.

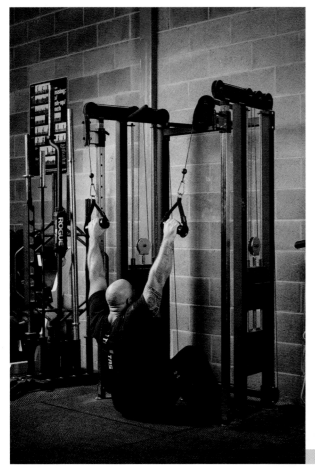
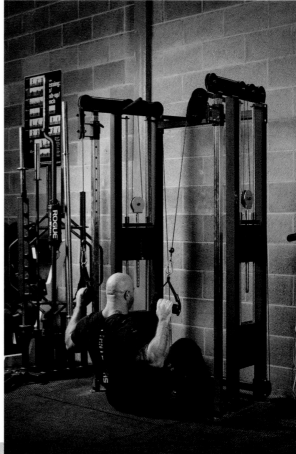

LAT PULL-DOWN

Pull-downs are a great way to develop and enhance vertical pulling strength, especially for heavier individuals who may achieve only a few pull-up reps per set. Cables can hit a similar movement pattern yet be loaded so that the individual can perform a high volume of reps and get the desired stimulus.

PERFECT FORM

- Take a grip that's slightly wider than shoulder width. If seated on the floor (as pictured), ensure you don't simply fall backwards to initiate the movement with your bodyweight. A rigid torso should be maintained at all times.
- Initiate the movement by retracting your shoulder blades, then continue it by bringing your elbows down to your sides until the bar is just below chin height.
- Squeeze the target muscles at the bottom of the move and avoid rocking back to assist the movement.
- Return to the start under control.

EXPERT TIP

I train both bilateral and unilateral versions of this to try to exhaust the full potential of the exercise. The mind-muscle connection is also vital to ensure that you retract the shoulder blades and get the most out of every rep.

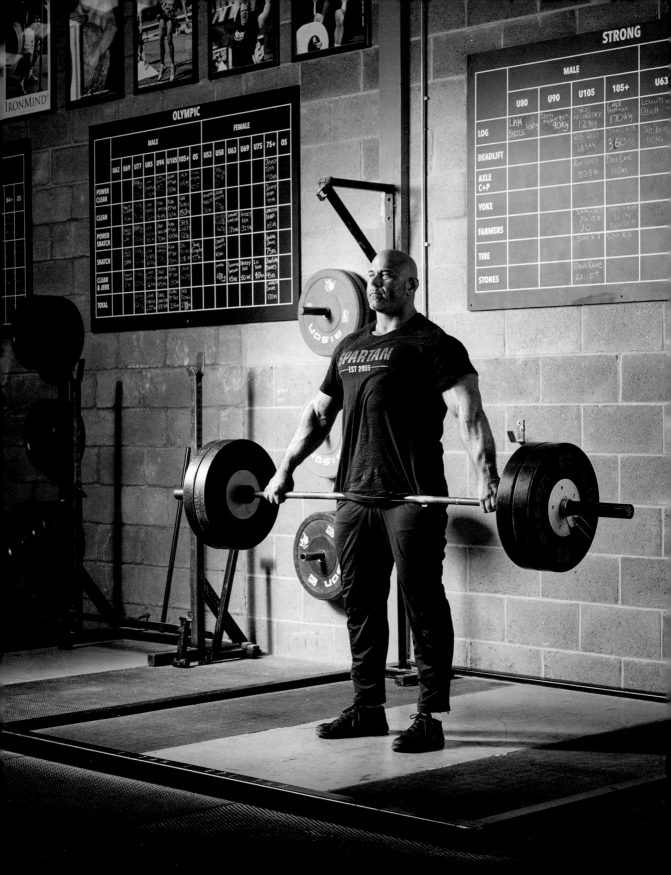

06.

PROGRAMME DESIGN

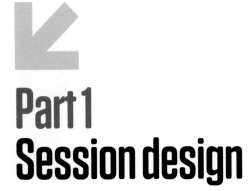

Part 1
Session design

By the time you read this, ideally you won't just have read through the book but implemented the tips and advice within it and worked your way through from the foundation section to the hypertrophy assistance lifts. You should be highly proficient in everything we've discussed – it's like you've graduated. But now that you can do the things I recommend and do them well, how do you put it all together?

This chapter is about making things practical. We've given you advice about how to do a squat; now it's time to apply that in your training. In this instance, we're going to look at how to apply the methods to a regular gym-goer, as opposed to a professional athlete. I also want to be clear that this book is about strength methods and that means it's about performance-based programming, whether you're an athlete or not.

There are two main areas that we're going to look at. First and foremost, using the information we've given you in the book, how you go about structuring a session. Second, how you go about structuring a training week and beyond.

In this section I've given you an outline of all of the components I include in a typical strength training session. This is a guide, not a list of commandments. What you put in these sessions should reflect what's right for the person doing them. The same goes for the typical training week. I've given you an outline of how you could structure the sessions, but you can adjust things to suit your needs.

Session breakdown
These are the main components of your strength training sessions

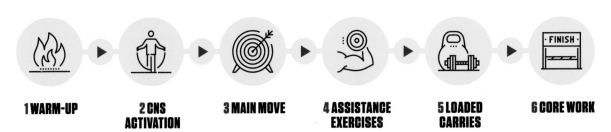

| 1 WARM-UP | 2 CNS ACTIVATION | 3 MAIN MOVE | 4 ASSISTANCE EXERCISES | 5 LOADED CARRIES | 6 CORE WORK |

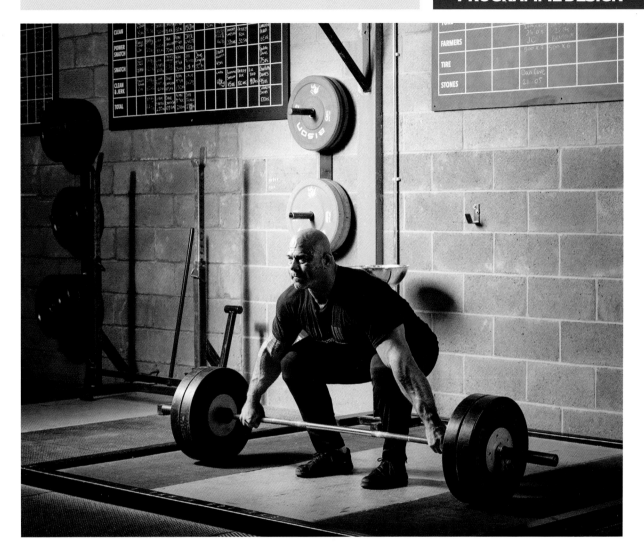

Once you've got a good understanding about how to construct a session, we turn to the idea of training cycles. Essentially, a cycle is a block of work with a specific purpose. We'll look at the three main types of cycles, starting with the shortest, which is also known as a microcycle, through to a mesocycle and finishing with a macrocycle, which is the largest of the training blocks.

As with the session breakdown, I've focused on what's most important, rather than trying to give you an exhaustive treatment of the subject. With this knowledge you can take charge of, rather than be overwhelmed by, the programming process.

Programme breakdown

These are the main components of your programmes, which are outlined on p168

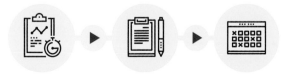

1 MICROCYCLE   **2 MESOCYCLE**   **3 MACROCYCLE**

COMPONENT 1

Warm-up

The first thing I think about when constructing a session is the warm-up or preparation phase. The key aims for a warm-up are to raise the core temperature, perform appropriate self-myofascial release (whether that's with a foam roller or a ball – it's essentially soft-tissue management) and mobility drills. The key thing with the myofascial release and the mobility drills performed within the warm-up period is that they should always be pertinent to the workout ahead.

As a starting point for general strength training, I advocate a minimum of four workouts per week. These workouts are comprised of key movement patterns. For example:

STRENGTH TRAINING FOUR-DAY SPLIT

DAY 1	Bench press and assistance
DAY 2	Deadlift and assistance
DAY 3	Overhead press and assistance
DAY 4	Squat and assistance

The assistance exercises on each day will be specific to and complement the main lift. Therefore, the warm-up for each session should be equally specific. Take the bench press as an example. If we look at what would be useful, what are the normal restrictions that people face when doing the bench press? It could be that they have tight lats. It could be that they've got tight pecs. It could be that they have poor shoulder mobility so maybe we need to release the shoulder capsule and perform shoulder mobility drills. We need to do anything we can to help them get into the correct position when they perform the bench press.

Ideally I'd spend five to ten minutes on this section. We want it to be brief. I could give you 15 things that would make a great warm-up. But the point is that this is a warm-up, not a workout, and that's a distinction you need to be clear about. If you look at some mobility experts on social media and you go through all of their drills, well, they'll take you 40 or 50 minutes. It's all valid, but we have a strength session to do so it's about getting the right amount done in minimal time. So you need to be judicious about your choices of movements.

In reality, the thing that might take the most time would be raising the core temperature and that could be done with something as simple as using an air bike or a rowing machine. If the individual is capable then it could be skipping. That might be 5-10 minutes alone, depending on the individual's needs. I'd say spend about 10-15 minutes max for the warm-up.

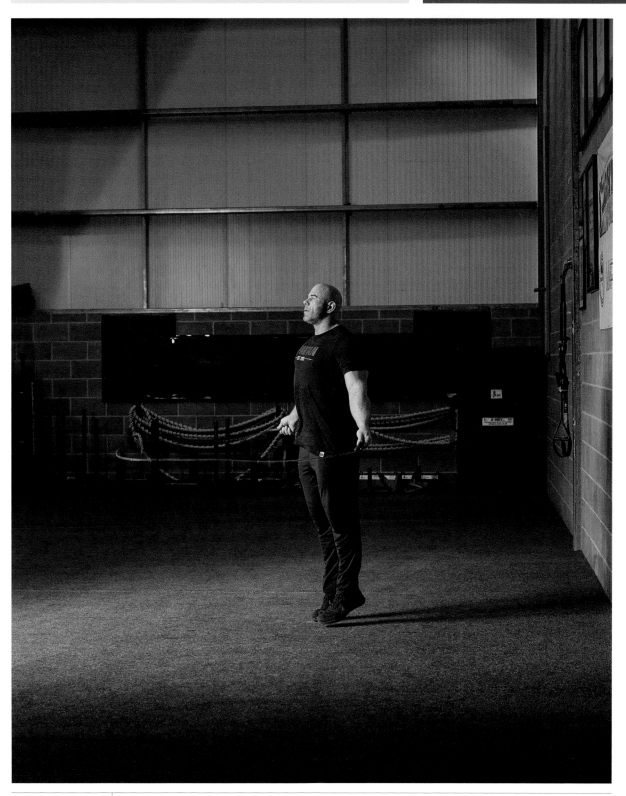

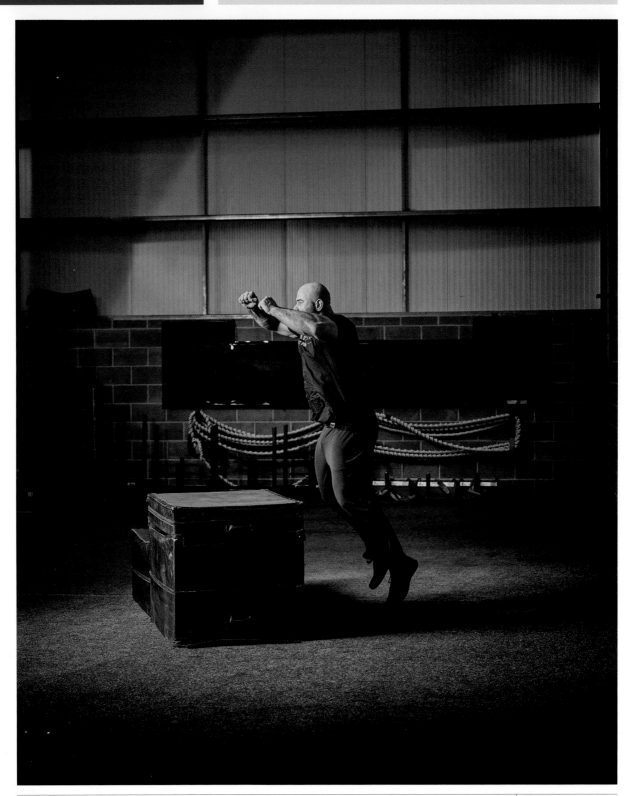

COMPONENT 2

CNS activation

This phase will enhance your power potential for the workout ahead. The jumps, throws and sprints in these drills will help you switch on to the session mentally as well as increasing your rate of force development. To me, it's almost like the world's best pre-workout. I demand maximal application from my clients for the session, but they may come to me stressed or tired, so we really need to help them get the most out of their session.

The specifics will vary depending on the individual. That's a key point worth mentioning. Someone could read through this book and become highly proficient only in the foundation exercises and the key barbell lifts. Those alone will increase power. Just increasing basic strength on the barbell will increase your rate of force development. That might be all that the individual needs, in which case the CNS activation drills will be very basic in nature and short in duration, and they'll be more focused on simply increasing mental stimulus.

However, a more advanced individual, perhaps with a few more training miles on the clock with the barbell, will require more specific drills. Someone who you could class as a novice – even if they've read the whole of this book – could use something as basic as skipping. It's a base plyometric. It's short and sweet. Or it could be something as simple as a medicine ball slam,

which increases rate of force development and really excites the nervous system. For someone with a bit more time under the bar I might include things like box jumps or even sprints. There are also some more advanced versions of medicine ball throws. It's about choosing the right exercise for the individual.

For CNS activation it's very much quality of movement over quantity that we're looking for. We want maximum application, whether that's a basic skipping exercise or a box jump. Whatever it is, every rep needs to be performed with maximum intensity. I like to use the term 'bad intentions'. We want them to be performed as aggressively as possible. We want them to recruit as many muscle fibres as possible. That's pretty demanding on the CNS, which means we're looking at low reps and quite possibly low sets as well with periods of complete rest in between. Just as we don't want to turn our the warm-up into a workout, we don't want to turn the CNS activation into a conditioning session.

When I say we want full rest, it's important to clarify that if you're doing box jumps, for example, you might do three sets of five reps with 60-90 seconds' rest in between. It's not going to be an epic amount of time. It would be completely different if this was a power development session for an athlete. That would run much longer.

COMPONENT 3

Main movement

When building a strength training programme, it's this move that we build the entire session around. The whole focus of the session is on improving our ability and performance in that particular movement. The chosen warm-up and CNS activation were both specific to this movement and, equally, anything that's going to follow the main strength movement is designed to complement it as well.

You obviously use the main movement as a means to get stronger but you also use it as a diagnostic tool to help with the assistance exercises. You can identify any weaknesses in the main lift and that should help with your choice of assistance exercises.

The main move is what we spend most time on and the higher the calibre of the lifter, the greater the number of warm-up sets required before you hit what are classed as working sets. If you're working up to a solid five reps and you can squat

100kg for five reps then your warm-up sets are going to be far fewer than someone who can perform five reps with 250kg.

I start every lift with an empty bar. A mistake I've made in the past is feeling like, if I'm training someone who can bench press 200kg, that I'm doing them a disservice to start with an empty bar. But that overlooks the fact that there's a very specific movement pattern which is a skill that we're trying to perform. That's something that I really want to emphasise – the ability to lift incredibly well. And every time I use an empty bar as a warm-up set, I'm greasing the groove to get that bar into the right bar path. It's not demanding on you physically and it's not like you're going to miss your target weight because you did an extra warm-up set with an empty bar.

You need to prepare yourself if you want to lift to the best of your ability. You've already freed yourself up with the warm-up. You've engaged yourself with the CNS activation. If you miss out those two steps, you'll still be able to squat and bench but you will not be able to squat and bench as well as you can. We can continue that positive preparation carryover with judicious use of warm-up sets. If we've got 20-30 reps before you're lifting a heavy weight then that's 20-30 reps where you're improving the muscles' ability to fire correctly. The more you practise that skill, the better position you're in to execute those skills under higher loads, which is ultimately where you want to be working. On the main lift we ideally want to be working in the 80% of one-rep max range and above.

The warm-up sets can be an effective tool but we don't want them to turn into a workout, so selecting the right number is part of the art of coaching. Everybody is different and everybody has a different training age. Some people

> **'You use the main movement as a means to get stronger, but you also use it as a diagnostic tool to identify any weaknesses'**

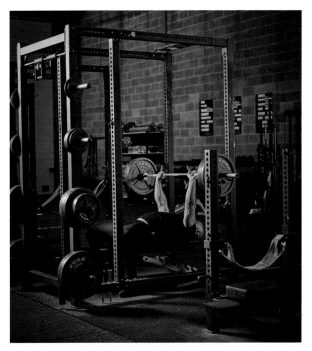

have been training for two years, some people for five years – but it may be that the person who has been training for five years has been training absolute dog shit, which means they actually have zero years experience of good-quality barbell training. That's one reason why how many warm-up sets you do has to vary from one individual to the next.

I have three clients that I'm working with. In each session each will be treated on an individual basis. In theory they can all lift and we're definitely going to be using a strength movement, but how many sets and reps I will use for warm-ups will be dictated by the individual. It could also be dictated by how fatigued they are when they come into the gym or maybe there's a negative carryover from the build-up from the rest of the week's training.

Let's say we're using the bench press. Typically I'd want anywhere between 3-5 warm-up sets then 3-5 working sets to hit the target weight that we're working towards. That means we're looking at between 6-10 total sets with adequate rest in between.

If I'm working with someone for whom I've identified an accurate one-rep max, then I like to use a percentage-based system and give them a specific target weight to hit at all times. It may be that we're working up to 4 sets of 3 reps at 80% of one-rep max. In that case, you know exactly how many kilograms 80% is. If 80% is 120kg then we know we've got to go from 20kg, the empty barbell, all the way up to 120kg.

Percentage-based training

EXAMPLE 1
In the first table, the individual's back squat 1RM has been identified as 200kg. The day's workout specifies 4 x 3 @ 80% of this 1RM. Therefore our target working weight is 4 x 3 @ 160kg.

EXAMPLE 2
If the individual had a back squat 1RM of 300kg and the workout parameters were the same (4 x 3 @ 80%) our warm-up would look like the second table.

SET	REPS	LOAD	TYPE
1	10	20kg	Warm-up
2	5	60kg	Warm-up
3	3	80kg	Warm-up
4	3	100kg	Warm-up
5	2	120kg	Warm-up
6	2	140kg	Warm-up
7	3	160kg	Work
8	3	160kg	Work
9	3	160kg	Work
10	3	160kg	Work

SET	REPS	LOAD	TYPE
1	10	20kg	Warm-up
2	5	60kg	Warm-up
3	5	100kg	Warm-up
4	3	140kg	Warm-up
5	3	180kg	Warm-up
6	3	200kg	Warm-up
7	2	215kg	Warm-up
8	1	230kg	Warm-up
9	4	240kg	Work
10	4	240kg	Work
11	4	240kg	Work
12	4	240kg	Work

Advanced
Daily Max method

For more advanced individuals, those further along on their strength training journey, I prefer a system called the Daily Max (DM) method. This entails working up to a technically sound single but NOT an all-time maximum weight – a weight that you could do two, possibly three reps with. Depending on the individual, their experience and condition on the day, I may want them to do two or three more singles with that weight, but that's a very small percentage of the training population.

The DM method enables you to lift to your maximum ability every single workout. From the DM you set on the day we would then perform our 'working sets' for reps at a set %, typically 80-90% of the daily max.

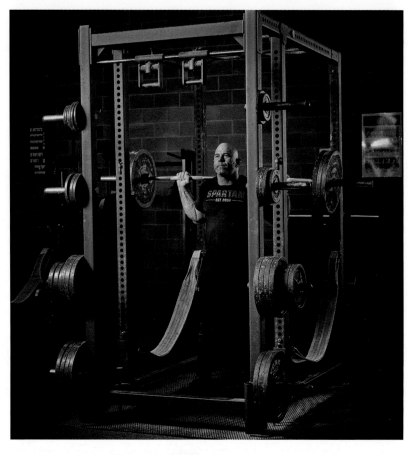

This is the exact workout I gave Dan Cave, a national champion 105kg strongman, on back squat. By using the DM method I was able to work him at 80% of his ability that very day, not some previous 1RM. Thus the stimulus was very specific. I find this method works incredibly well with powerlifters and strongmen and strongwomen.

STEP 1 Identify back squat DM based on ability that day

SET	REPS	LOAD	TYPE
1	10	20kg	Warm-up
2	5	80kg	Warm-up
3	5	100kg	Warm-up
4	3	140kg	Warm-up
5	2	180kg	Warm-up
6	1	220kg	Warm-up
7	1	260kg	Warm-up
8	1	300kg	Warm-up
9	1	310kg	Warm-up

STEP 2 Complete work sets for that day

SET	REPS	LOAD	TYPE
1	4	250kg	Work
2	4	250kg	Work
3	4	250kg	Work
4	4	250kg	Work
5	4	250kg	Work

Inexperienced
Rep Max system

For those newer to strength training a percentage-based system is not always the best option. Often times these people are unable to set an accurate one-rep max (1RM) from which to identify working percentages – either because they lack the confidence to handle maximum weights, or because they are unable to maintain excellent form under higher loads. In this case I simply have them work up each day to a Rep Max (RM) in the 3-5 rep range. That means basically the heaviest weight they can handle with perfect form for between 3 and 5 reps. Each subsequent week they aim to improve on this number.

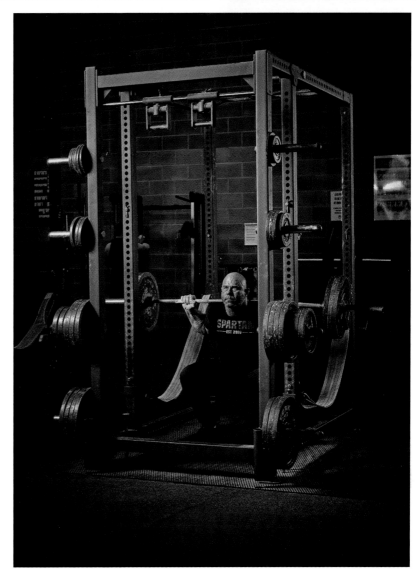

This is another back squat example. The target for the day is 5 technically sound reps with the heaviest weight possible, without failing a rep or seeing their form break down.

SET	REPS	LOAD	TYPE
1	10	20kg	Warm-up
2	5	40kg	Warm-up
3	5	60kg	Warm-up
4	5	80kg	Warm-up
5	5	90kg	Warm-up
6	5	95kg	Work

The objective here would be to ideally get 97.5kg x 5 in the following week's session.

This method works very well for those new to strength training and whose strength will jump week to week with relative ease. So the majority of the time, I'm simply thinking about getting people strong in the 3-5 rep range. Gradually over time I would cycle down from 5RM to 3RM and ultimately 1RM when ready.

Once a reliable 1RM can be identified I prefer to switch to a percentage-based programme.

Perfect form

Regardless of the loading system I always want technically perfect reps. Not do-or-die reps. I never want someone to perform a rep where there's a breakdown in technique. It's a slower approach but strength training is a long-term project. I don't see any benefit to any athlete by performing a dodgy rep.

After I write this, I'm working with three top-end strength athletes today, culminating with the World's Strongest Woman, Donna Moore. Everything they lift today will be technically perfect and there are two main reasons for that. If you allow sloppy reps then that makes a lack of discipline acceptable. And if you're not using perfect form you're settling for an 80% result. If I'm working with a powerlifter, that's not going to pass in a powerlifting competition. So, yeah, you might have got a great gym lift that can go on Instagram but that athlete is only judged by how they perform on the platform. So what use is a dodgy rep? It's no use.

When you perform the lifts in the foundation section of this book, I want them to look effortless. Your pull-ups, press-ups, kettlebells swings –they should all look perfect. You don't need to see veins popping out of the forehead. I want to see technically perfect movements. When you move on to the main barbell lifts you'll eventually get strong enough to be lifting sufficient weight so that you really have to fight to lift the weight perfectly. That's

fine. But if it becomes a grinder of a rep, that is incredibly costly to the central nervous system, which will have a negative impact on the rest of the session and possibly even the next session.

I respect tenacity and fight but I'd be failing in my job if I was to encourage a client to go for a rep that I knew they were going to fail. Don't get me wrong, there's a time and a place for utter commitment to the cause where you simply have to go above and beyond to achieve a result, especially when we're looking at hypertrophy methods where we're trying to induce as much muscle trauma as possible to then stimulate and encourage a growth response. But I do not put those same conditions on strength training. I want you to perform your strength training reps like an Olympic lifter. I want technical perfection.

You've got to be smart with how you train. It's so easy to get carried away and judge the quality of a session by how physically destroyed you are. You've probably heard of the 20-rep squat protocol. Well, you could do that. And you could put bands on the bar to make it harder. And you could make someone pause for 10 seconds at the bottom of each rep to make it even harder. It's very easy to make something as painful and as torturous as possible. But is that the optimal way to get the result you want? Almost never.

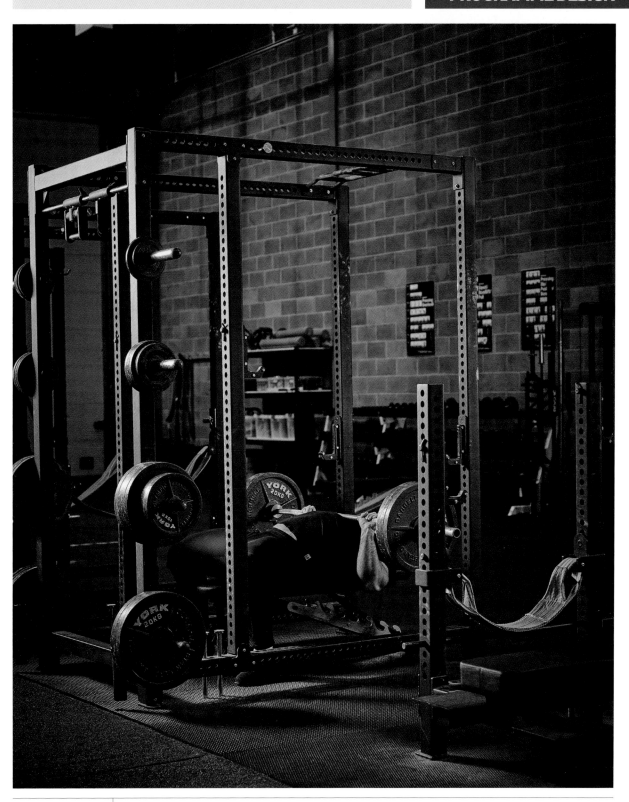

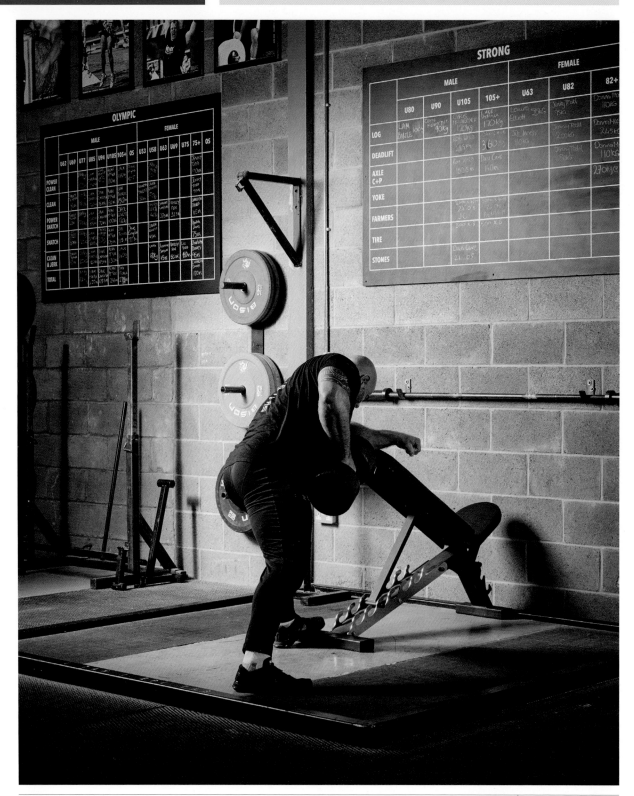

COMPONENT 4

Assistance exercises

As we've seen, the main lift can identify weaknesses, and those weaknesses can then be addressed and strengthened with assistance work. But we can also use assistance exercises to increase hypertrophy. The way I look at it, muscle is like armour. When it comes to strength training, I want to put as much armour on my clients as possible because a bigger muscle has a greater potential to be a stronger muscle. As well as that, we can use assistance work to help develop muscular endurance and work capacity. So there's an enormous amount of value in the assistance lifts because they can address so many different aspects at the same time.

How many assistance moves you use will be dictated by the weaknesses that you exhibit in the main lift. I'll give you an example. Let's say we're looking at the squat. Now, this is a strength training programme, remember. Let's say that the individual concerned is able to perform a technically sound squat but once they start hitting the higher percentages – say 85% and above – they start to tip forwards. If we're assuming it's not a technique flaw, what does it suggest? We're looking at a strength leak in the torso. So maybe the assistance exercise should be a pause squat, where you're pausing for three to five seconds at the base of a squat to strengthen torso rigidity and strength out of the hole.

It could be that they're deadlifting and they're weak from the floor to the mid-shin. In that case, maybe we employ deficit deadlifts. The weakness could even be in their lats in which case we may prescribe paused snatch-grip deadlifts. We could exaggerate the lowering, eccentric phase and play with the tempo. There are many options, but the key is in being able to accurately identify the correct weakness.

I'm likely to pick between one and three assistance movements that are specific to the main lift. There's no hard and fast answer but I normally prefer four sets of anywhere between four and eight reps. You need to use an appreciable load to get strong but you don't want to go too high on reps because you'd sacrifice the load that you can carry as fatigue sets in. Equally, you don't want to go too low on reps because then the load will be too heavy.

You can also bring in hypertrophy methods so, if we take the deadlift, it would certainly benefit the lifter to have more developed hamstrings, glutes and quads. For that you're looking at anywhere between eight and 20 reps. And I'm thinking about exercises such as hamstring curls and split squats. They won't necessarily address the strength leak in the main lift. We've already dealt with that. But we're adding muscle and we can even develop muscular endurance and work capacity too.

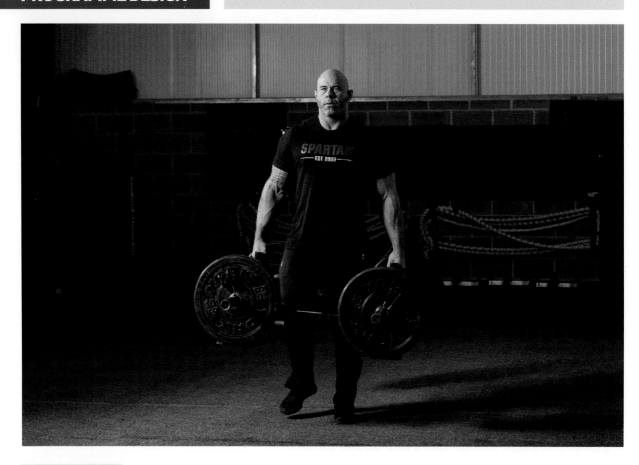

COMPONENT 5
Loaded carries

You'll notice that I put loaded carries before core. Of course, a loaded carry is a core exercise, which allows us to have a great training economy, should we need it. So it may be that I won't do loaded carries and core-specific exercises in the same workout. What I'm giving you is a sample structure of a session with every facet that can be included.

You might have done two assistance exercises to address a weakness in the main lift and then a superset for hypertrophy so you may be short on time. If that's the case, my go-to for core work is loaded carries. I'd much rather include loaded carries in every single session than squeeze some traditional core work in.

A loaded carry will address strength leaks in the main lift but on top of that they will work the grip, they'll work the mind and they're a great metabolic conditioner. They're great for building muscle, burning fat – they do everything.

On a squat day, for example, you've got the option of sleds, prowlers or maybe even a yoke. On bench press day you've got loaded carries, overhead carries or Zercher carries. There are so many options but the key reason to include them, as I said in the loaded carries chapter, is that they do so many things. I'm yet to come across a client who wouldn't benefit from doing loaded carries.

If you're familiar with the Pallof press, it looks awesome if you take the right pictures. And you could write a really good article about why you should do them that would make you look like you know what you're talking about. But I will choose a Zercher carry ten times out of ten over a Pallof press. Yes, there's a benefit to the Pallof press but there's a much greater return from correctly executed loaded carries. Granted, if I'm working with an injured person or someone who just cannot perform certain carries then I won't use them. But generally the benefits are just so high.

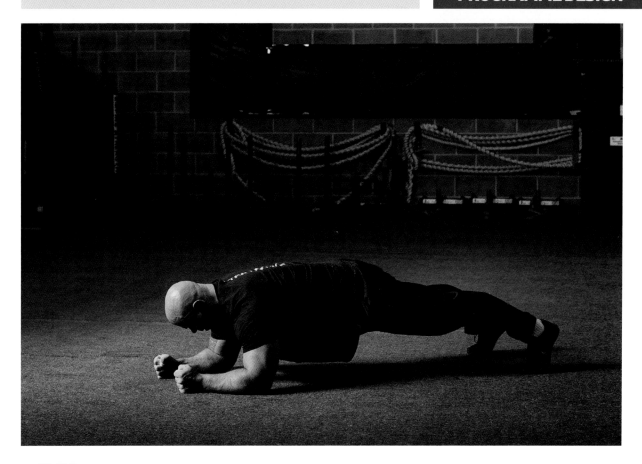

COMPONENT 6

Core work

Core training can be performed at any point throughout the workout and I like to focus on the 'McGill Big 3', a set of exercises recommended by Dr Stuart McGill. Basically, it's three movements – a McGill sit-up, a bird-dog and a McGill side plank – and they are all ways to increase rigidity through the torso. If you perform those exercises then your brace will be stronger in the remainder of the session. They can be used in the warm-up section to facilitate greater performance by improving your ability to brace and to maintain the brace in the main lift. For the sake of economy, we could use them as active rest fillers but we never want to detract from the main lifts in the sessions.

I'm reluctant to thoughtlessly tack on core-specific exercises to the end of the session. You see it all the time, you know – 'I'll throw in three sets of ten leg raises in at the end of a session just for the hell of it'. But you know fine well that the things you do at the end of a workout aren't going to get the same level of intensity

as the things that you do at the start of the workout. It's about being smart, and I'm looking for exercises that will strengthen the link between breathing, bracing and maintaining a position under load – things that we've been talking about from the start of this book. So if we've implemented some of the McGill Big 3 in the warm-up, we've already had direct core work that way, then we've got loaded carries, which have a direct core stimulus. So any extra core work would be specific to the individual. If you have a weakness in any of those areas then you may look to address it.

From a strength training perspective, why am I trying to make the core stronger? It's not so I can look good with my top off, although that's a side effect of smart training and good nutritional habits. What's far more important for me is that your midsection can perform the way it is supposed to in order to facilitate the main strength lift so that you have a bulletproof physique.

Sample sessions

The sample sessions over the following pages have been set out to give you an idea about how I would construct a session for each of the four main strength training lifts: the bench press, the deadlift, the squat and the overhead press. I've used a different training phase for each lift to give you an insight into how the stage you're at in your programme will affect the main training variables. To find more information about the main training phases turn to p168.

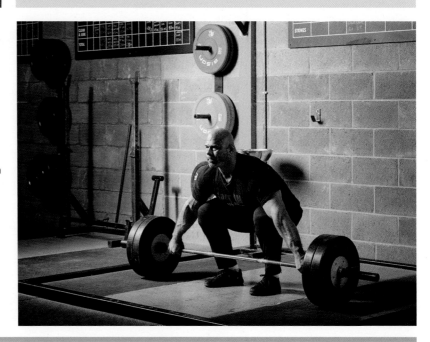

Warm-up

COMPONENT	EXERCISE	ACTIVITY	NOTES
Raise core temp	Air bike or row	5-10min	Aim to burn roughly 50-100 calories.
Self-myofascial release	**Deadlift or squat day:** lats, glutes, hip flexors, hamstrings and quads **Press day (bench and overhead):** lats, pecs and thoracic spine	1-3min each area	
Mobility	**Deadlift or squat day:** lower body drills **Press day (bench and overhead):** upper body drills	10-15 reps per exercise	On deadlift and squat day I like to add 3-5 sets of 10-20 reps of terminal knee extensions and light hamstring curls. On pressing days I like to add 3-5 sets of 10-20 reps of upper back/scapular retraction movements such as face pulls and band pull-aparts.
CNS activation	**Deadlift day:** med ball scoop throw or slam, or explosive Russian kettlebell swing **Bench day:** plyo press-up (from incline bench, flat bench or floor) **Squat day:** box jump **Press day:** med ball push press throw	3-5 sets of 3-5 reps with 75sec rest between exercises on all days	

Bench press workout (accumulation phase)

COMPONENT	EXERCISE	SETS	REPS	REST	NOTES
Main lift	Bench press	-	-	120sec	Sets and reps determined by using percentage, Daily Max or Rep Max systems described on p155-157.
Assistance 1	Dumbbell bench press	4	6-8	90-120sec	Strengthen weak area in main lift.
Assistance 2	Floor press	4	6-8	90-120sec	Strengthen weak area in main lift.
Hypertrophy	Cable triceps press-down	3	8-12	75-90sec	

Deadlift workout (intensification phase)

COMPONENT	EXERCISE	SETS	REPS	REST	NOTES
Main lift	Deadlift	-	-	120sec	Sets and reps determined by using percentage, Daily Max or Rep Max systems described on p155-157.
Assistance 1	Deficit deadlift	4	6-8	90-120sec	Strengthen weak area in main lift.
Assistance 2	Deadlift from blocks	4	6-8	90-120sec	Lift from just below the knees. Create an overload and handle heavier load.
Hypertrophy	Pull-up or chin-up	3	10-12	75-90sec	You could superset the two hypertrophy exercises for both time and training effect.
	Glute/ham raise, 45 raise, reverse hyperextension, glute bridge or hip thrust	3	10-12	75-90sec	
Loaded carry	Farmer's walk	4	20m	120sec	

Overhead press workout (realisation phase)

COMPONENT	EXERCISE	SETS	REPS	REST	NOTES
Main lift	Military press	–	–	120sec	Sets and reps determined by using percentage, Daily Max or Rep Max systems described on p155-157.
Assistance 1	Push press	4	6-8	90-120sec	Maximise your strength.
Assistance 2	Military press from pins	4	6-8	90-120sec	Set the pins at forehead height. Create an overload and handle heavier load.
Hypertrophy	Delts or triceps exercise	3	12-15	75-90sec	

Squat workout (intensification phase)

COMPONENT	EXERCISE	SETS	REPS	REST	NOTES
Main lift	Back squat	–	–	120sec	Sets and reps determined by using percentage, Daily Max or Rep Max systems described on p155-157.
Assistance 1	Paused back squat	4	6-8	90-120sec	Strengthen weak area in main lift.
Assistance 2	Front squat	4	6-8	90-120sec	Strengthen weak area in main lift.
Hypertrophy	Leg press	3	8-12	75-90sec	
Loaded carry	Log Zercher carry	4	20m	90-120sec	

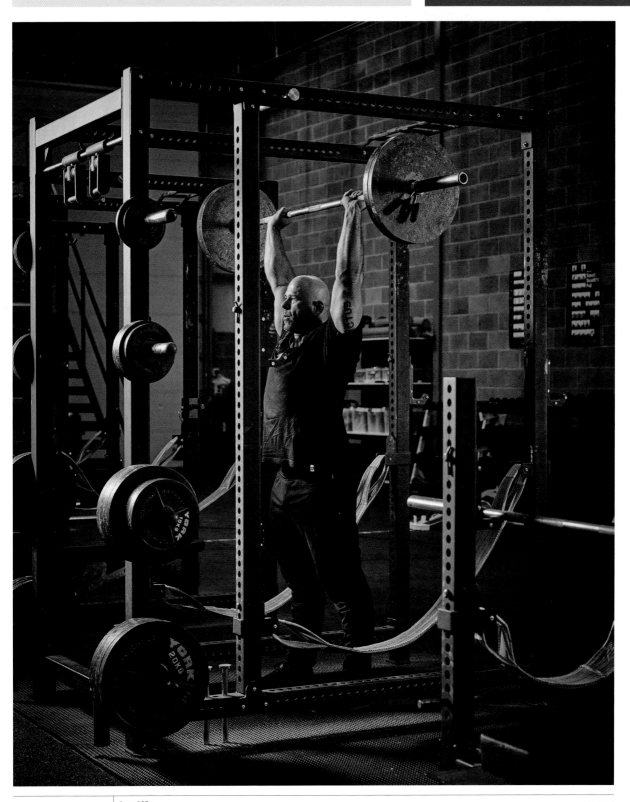

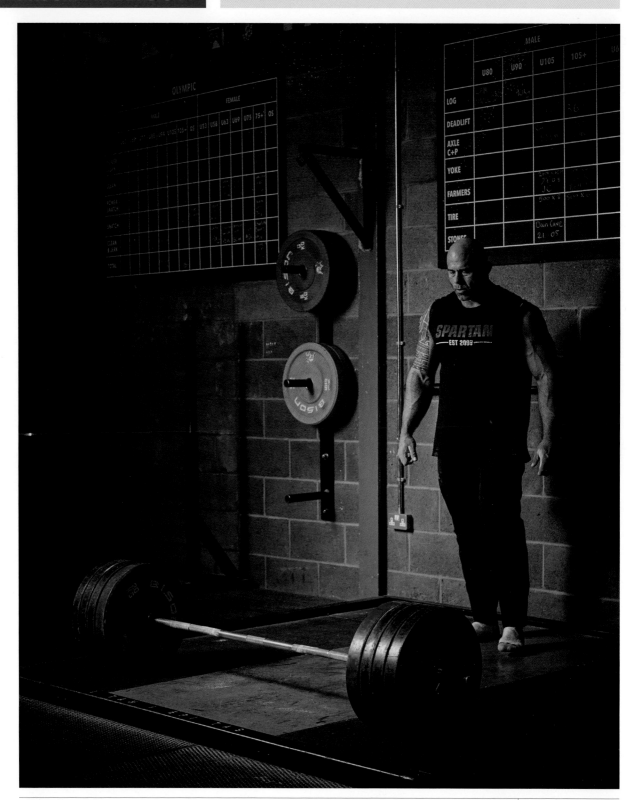

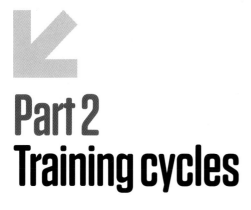

Part 2
Training cycles

I always advocate training with a specific goal in mind. And the best way to get to that endpoint is to have a programme. In my experience, it's easier to break your overall goal down into short-term, medium-term and long-term goals. The short-term goals add up to achieving the medium-term goals and the medium-term goals add up to achieving the long-term goal. That's why we use training cycles, which are blocks of varying length known as microcycles, mesocycles and macrocycles. This section will help you to programme your cycles once you have identified your goal.

PHASE	DESCRIPTION
Microcycle	7 days minimum. Typically, one week with a focus on one specific goal.
Mesocycle	Typically 4-6 weeks to achieve a certain goal. I tend to break these mesocycles down into accumulation, intensification and realisation phases.
Macrocycle	Typically at least 12 weeks, working towards a yearly goal or longer – for example, Olympic athletes have macrocycles that last four years.

Microcycle structure

You now know how to put a session together, but how would that session fit into a week?

I'm going to set this out with someone who is training with the priority of strength and performance. Yes, they may want to have a bit more muscle mass and this will elicit that, to an extent. But the priority is building strength.

Another caveat that I need to mention is that this structure works best when you commit fully to the cause so that every single session is performed to the highest possible level. I want maximum results and that requires a maximum effort investment, and maximum application at all times.

What we've got here is a tremendous starting point that will improve your strength with the key lifts. You can address your weaknesses with the assistance exercises. You can build an appreciable amount of muscle by using hypertrophy methods with the assistance exercises. And you can become a bit of a fucking god on the loaded carries. On top of that, if you can get your nutrition and sleep on point, then the world is your oyster and you've got so many training avenues that you can explore.

This system will work for 52 weeks of the year. Yes, you can shoot off and use some super deadlift programme for four weeks that will make your deadlift shoot up. That's great. But that's a flash in the pan. It'll make a big jump but then it stalls. This is your default mechanism for long-term sustained progress.

The general structure rule I would go with – provided increased strength is the aim – is a minimum of four training sessions per week. We could drop down to three sessions a week if it was an absolute necessity. I could also increase to five or six sessions a week if it was warranted. The only exceptions may be athletes such as MMA fighters or rugby players who may only have enough time to complete two good-quality strength training sessions a week. But for general-population clients I wouldn't go lower than three sessions a week.

I'm wary of speaking in absolutes but all I can genuinely say is that, if strength is the goal, then as a starting point, this is the most effective way that I've found of dividing up a week. It's something that Canadian coach, and my mentor, Christian Thibaudeau teaches, and it's something that I buy into.

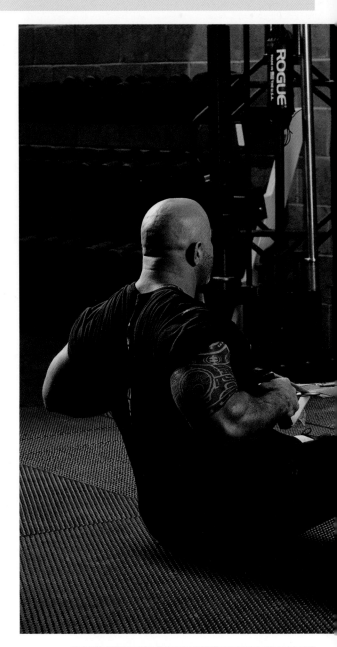

TRAINING WEEK RULES

1 Four training sessions per week

2 Never train more than two days in a row

3 Never have more than one rest day in a row

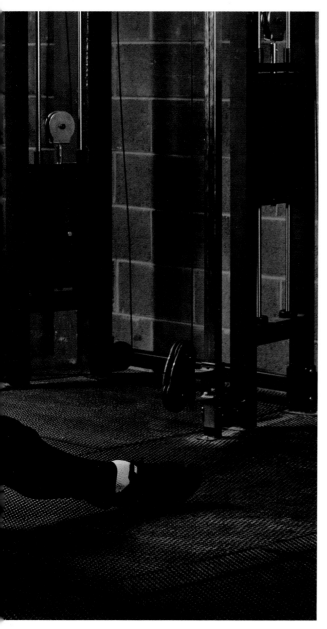

In my gym, this is ideally where I start a client who has graduated through all of the lifts in this book so I can see what they are capable of doing. It's also about what they can recover from. Of course maximum application every session is required, but they need to be able to recover so they can grow and come back stronger, ready to apply themselves fully in the next session.

If an individual rests more than one day in a row I find that performance drops. I find that if people have both Saturday and Sunday off they are more sluggish when the Monday session comes around. It's like they get out of the training groove.

I also find that this structure is good for client adherence. If I'm seeing someone for four sessions a week, that's only four hours out of 168 in the week. But where do you think the real changes are going to be happening? They're not with me. It's what they do with their lifestyle, their nutrition – everything they do when they're not with me – that's going to make the difference. So if I've got a new client who likes to go off the rails at the weekend, giving them both Saturday and Sunday off probably won't help. But the chances are that their nutrition will be better before and after a training session.

I can attest to this personally. I don't train on a Sunday and that is the diciest day for me nutrition wise because I don't have as much structure to my day. It's a relaxed day but it's like my foot is off the gas. The reality is that we're all human and we're all fallible. With my clients, the days they have a session at Spartan Performance are more structured and there's a greater chance of them following both an optimal nutrition and recovery plan.

For most people, myself included, starting the training week on a Monday tends to be both the most practical and effective. **REST DAYS** These should be every non-strength training day shown in the table on the right. Always some form of low-intensity steady state (LISS) active recovery, such as walking, airbike, swim, sauna or mobility.

SAMPLE TRAINING WEEK

Option	MON	TUE	WED	THUR	FRI	SAT	SUN
1	S1	Rest	S2	Rest	S3	S4	Rest
2	S1	S2	Rest	S3	Rest	S4	Rest
3	Rest	S1	Rest	S2	S3	Rest	S4

Main movement breakdown

The simplest way to break down the four training days is by individual movements. That means I have a squat day with appropriate assistance, I have a bench press day with appropriate assistance, I have a deadlift day with appropriate assistance and I have an overhead press day with appropriate assistance. If you want to get stronger then you're going to need to devote time to the key barbell lifts. That's why each session in the week is built around one of the big lifts.

A key thing that you need to be aware of is that I don't want something you do in session 1 to negatively affect something you do in session 2. So if you do bench press on Monday then you won't do overhead press on Tuesday because there will be a negative carryover from the pressing movements and the assistance moves you did on the bench press day.

SAMPLE TRAINING WEEK	
MON	Overhead press and assistance
TUE	Squat and assistance
WED	Rest and active recovery
THUR	Bench press and assistance
FRI	Rest and active recovery
SAT	Deadlift and assistance
SUN	Rest and active recovery

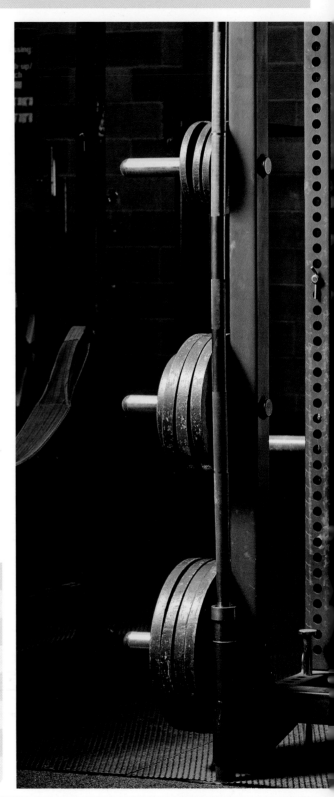

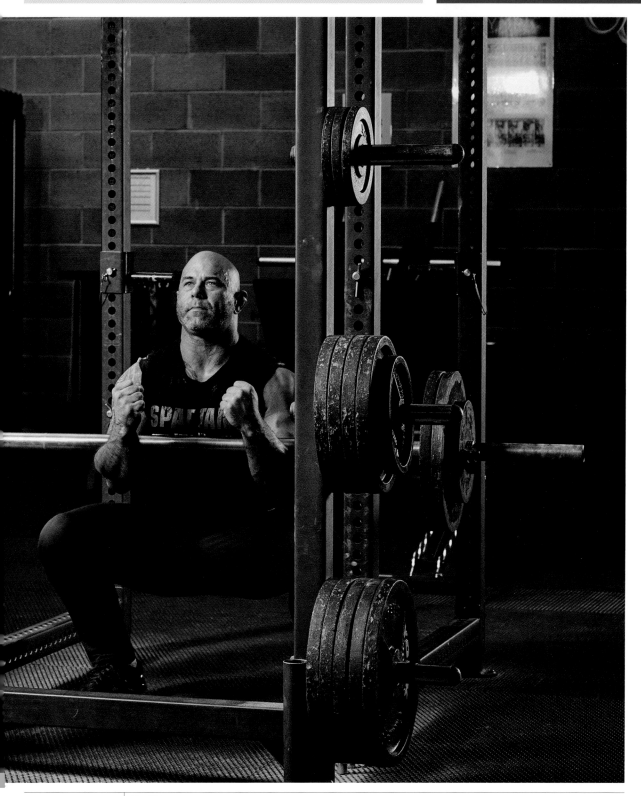

Three training sessions per week structure

Despite my preference for a minimum of four training sessions a week, I also live in the real world and acknowledge the demands on people's time. If I can get someone to have three incredible sessions a week, that's far better than overcommitting to four where they tend to make three and it's hit and miss whether they make the fourth session, and if they do the session it's short or rushed. So it's about what's best for the individual. You'll be able to achieve more in both the short and long term if you can do four days but only if that structure's optimal for the individual client.

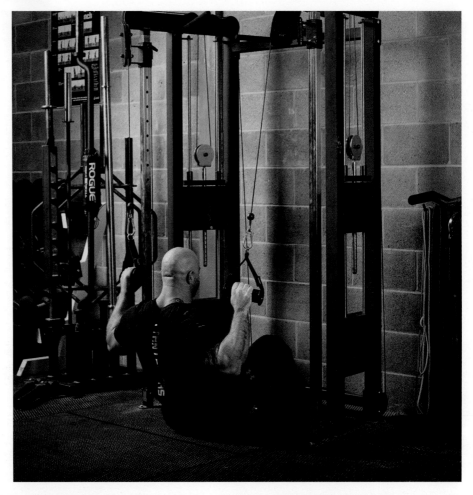

If we go down to three days a week we also have to change the structure of each session. I tend to go with two options here:
OPTION 1 Three days of full-body training over a seven-day training week.
OPTION 2 Adopt a nine-day training week as opposed to seven, where the fourth movement is performed on day 1 of week 2.

OPTION 1 SEVEN-DAY TRAINING WEEK	
MON	Squat and full-body assistance
TUE	Rest and active recovery
WED	Bench press and full-body assistance
THUR	Rest and active recovery
FRI	Deadlift and full-body assistance
SAT	Rest and active recovery
SUN	Rest and active recovery

OPTION 2 NINE-DAY TRAINING WEEK	
MON	Squat and full-body assistance
TUE	Rest and active recovery
WED	Bench press and full-body assistance
THUR	Rest and active recovery
FRI	Deadlift and full-body assistance
SAT	Rest and active recovery
SUN	Rest and active recovery
MON	Overhead press and full-body assistance
TUE	Rest and active recovery

Five training sessions per week structure

The deciding factor about whether or not I push someone up to five sessions a week is simple. Can they give me seven to nine hours' good-quality sleep a night? Are they adhering to the nutritional guidelines that I advocate 90% of the time? Because by adding an extra session you're adding extra stress. There's no point adding the extra stimulus and stress if the recovery methods aren't in place. Without adequate recovery you can get ill more frequently, pick up avoidable injuries or just lose interest.

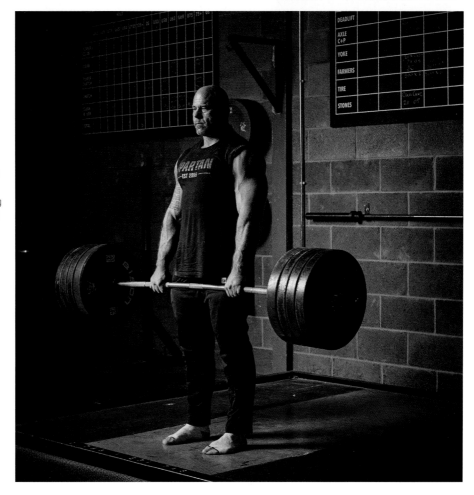

OPTION 1 This is the variation I use most frequently, where the fifth day focuses on direct arm, calf and core training.

OPTION 2 This time we use the fifth day to address key weaknesses even further. Most often this is a lack of posterior chain development (lower back, glutes and hamstrings).

OPTION 1 SAMPLE TRAINING WEEK

MON	Overhead press and assistance
TUE	Squat and assistance
WED	Bench press and assistance
THUR	Rest and active recovery
FRI	Deadlift and assistance
SAT	Biceps, calves and abs
SUN	Rest and active recovery

OPTION 2 SAMPLE TRAINING WEEK

MON	Squat and assistance
TUE	Overhead press and assistance
WED	Rest and active recovery
THUR	Deadlift and assistance
FRI	Bench press and assistance
SAT*	Posterior chain or pulling
SUN	Rest and active recovery

*I use this day to get some more volume in from movements such as Olympic lift variations, swings, 45 raises, glute/ham raises, glute bridges and hip thrusts.

It can also be a dedicated pulling day for greater back development. Lats in particular are important in deadlift, Olympic lift and overhead pressing strength.

Sample 13-week macrocycle

WEEKS 1-4 ACCUMULATION PHASE

The aim in this phase is to accumulate work and volume in the 80% range of your one-rep max. So you might start by doing five sets of three reps and progress to five sets of five reps by adding one rep per week. It's all about getting used to performing a lift in that range and not dropping the intensity.

For the assistance exercises, I use both of these to iron out a specific weakness. So, for example, if someone has a weak trunk and is tipping forwards when they're coming up out of the hole in the squat, I may tell them to use a paused back squat.

WEEKS 5-8 INTENSIFICATION PHASE

You've built a solid base so now we increase the intensity. The aim is to build up from 85-90% with a target of doing three sets of three reps in your main lift at 90%.

For the assistance moves we slightly adjust the focus. One focuses on strengthening a weakness, because you won't have ironed out all your weaknesses in the previous four weeks. The other is there to provide overload for the muscle, so you'd use a load that's greater than your 1RM for the main move – a half squat, for example. The loaded carry move is more in the strength range, in line with our overall training aim.

ELEMENT	NOTES
Intensity	Accumulate work in the 80% of 1RM range.
Main lift	Target is 4-5 sets of 4-6 reps at 80% of your 1RM.
Assistance	2 assistance exercises that address weakness identified in the main lift, performed in the 4-6 rep range.
Hypertrophy	1-2 hypertrophy movements, performed as 2-3 sets of 8-12 reps, to build the muscles. Main lifts focus on the capacity to use said muscles.
Extras	Loaded carry on squat and deadlift days. Performed for hypertrophy: minimum distance 40m, maximum distance 80m, ideal distance 60m.

ELEMENT	NOTES
Intensity	Main lift intensity increases to work in the 85%-90% range.
Main lift	Target is 3 sets of 3 reps at 90% of your 1RM by week 8.
Assistance	2 assistance exercises, one to strengthen a weakness and the other to create overload and better handle heavier loads, both performed as 4 sets of 4-6 reps.
Hypertrophy	1-2 hypertrophy movements, performed as 2-3 sets of 10-12 reps, to build the muscles. Main lifts focus on the capacity to use said muscles.
Extras	Loaded carry on squat and deadlift days. Performed for strength: minimum distance 10m, maximum distance 60m, ideal distance 20-40m.

WEEKS 9-12 REALISATION PHASE

You've done eight weeks of hard work. You've built a foundation, you've increased the intensity and now you want to realise your newfound strength. You're working in the 95-100% range for your main lift – a load that would have been too much in week 1 – and you are aiming to do your old 1RM for reps.

The assistance exercises are aimed at maximising strength so you're overloading your muscles where they are strongest. You want to capitalise on the strength you already have and create further overload. The hypertrophy and loaded carry components continue in line with the progression of the plan.

WEEK 13 PEAKING PHASE (OPTIONAL)

This is where you set your new 1RM. If I'm training the average Joe, I don't really see the need for this phase. I only tend to use it with athletes who complete in strength sports. For them, it's useful for a couple of reasons: they need to have an accurate 1RM and they also need to practise the skill of lifting heavy singles. The general population don't really need that and can calculate their new 1RM by using an online calculator. I also like people to train rather than being constantly tested, particularly if they are relatively new to training.

ELEMENT	NOTES
Intensity	Main lift intensity increases to work in the 95%-100% range.
Main lift	Target is 2-3 sets of 3 reps at 100% of your 1RM by week 8.
Assistance	2 assistance exercises, one to maximise strength and the other to create further overload, both performed as 4 sets of 4-6 reps.
Hypertrophy	1 hypertrophy movement, performed as 2-3 sets of 12-15 reps, to build the muscles. Main lifts focus on the capacity to use said muscles.
Extras	Loaded carry on squat and deadlift days. Performed for strength: minimum distance 10m, maximum distance 20m.

NOTES
Only complete this phase if you are setting or testing a new 1RM
Remove the assistance lifts to focus solely on the main lift.
I tend to reserve this for strength sports based individuals, such as powerlifters, weightlifters and strongman competitors, rather than using it with general population clients.

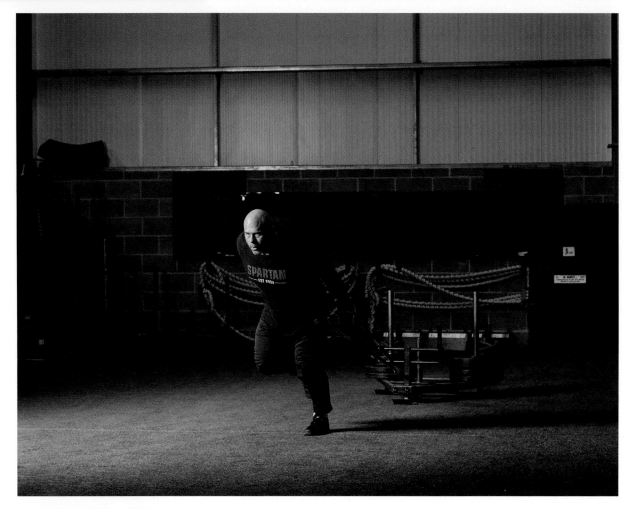

PROGRAMMING FAQ

Can I train too much?

You do get people who feel like they need to train every day. I admit I'm one of those people. I am a training addict. If I could train seven days a week, twice a day, I would. Not only is it my routine, it's part of my identity too. You could even class it as my therapy. So I appreciate the enthusiasm to train more, but it has to be reined in sometimes.

My clients have to earn the right to strength train more than four days a week because just adding an extra session does not guarantee that your strength gains will increase. You could add a session that ticks a box because you like doing it, but your results could drop. In that instance, what you're doing outside of the gym needs more attention. So as much as I'd like to indulge someone's desire to train more, I have to take a step back as a coach and ask, what are we training for? What is the goal? And is this person doing everything they can to recover optimally?

If you're desperate to lift every day, it's worth remembering that I encourage all my clients to train seven days a week – and what I mean by that is I want my clients to be physically active every single day. So whatever split you're on – three, four or five days – you must be proactive with your recovery on the days that you're not strength training.

We've got mobility routines that take 20-30 minutes that would get a good sweat on and might satisfy the desire to get a training stimulus without the need for a full session. They're also conducive to recovering between sessions. I also give clients the option of having an infra-red sauna or some soft tissue work with the physiotherapist. It could even be that I advise them to go and have a nice meal. The takeaway is that you should train hard but recover even harder. Of course, don't forget you must first train hard enough to have something to recover from! It works both ways.

How do I bring up lagging lifts?

Before I go into how I would address lagging lifts it's worth reiterating that I would set up the four-day split I've given as an example on the assumption that the individual is a graduate of the theory within this book. That would mean that they have the technical expertise to perform all of the lifts to a high standard. So if they're really struggling with one of the four key lifts they need to go back and work on the foundation section until they are sufficiently proficient to progress.

If someone is struggling in one of the key movements then we find the variations of that movement they can do while addressing the reasons why they're struggling with the key movement. If their limitation with the overhead press is due to shoulder mobility, say, then they can still train overhead pressing qualities and overhead strength while doing a one-arm landmine press. In my gym we have a pentagon bar press, which means you can do a landmine press with two hands. Landmine and pentagon presses fill a comfortable gap between a horizontal (bench) and vertical (overhead) press. So in that instance the overhead press day becomes a landmine press day as the main strength lift, but a lot of time within that session would be spent working on mobility to enable you to press vertically in the near future.

As well as that, the assistance would be specific to their weaknesses. They could also do an incline dumbbell bench press on a high incline. It wouldn't be as good as a standing dumbbell military press but if they don't have the ability to maintain the correct torso position then they can use a high incline position on the bench. So even if they have a weakness they can still improve overhead pressing strength and it's just a question of finding the right exercise and the right angle for the individual. After all, what is a coach? We're problem-solvers – because you rarely get people who fit into the perfect template with zero issues.

It could be that they are spot-on at squatting, benching and overhead press but their deadlift is the biggest issue. I'll use myself as a case in point. I struggled recently at conventional deadlifting from the floor with optimal technique but if I put the bar on a one-inch mat it was in the perfect position for me. Essentially my hamstring mobility wasn't optimal and I couldn't maintain a tight back under heavy loads. So if you can't perform a textbook lift there's always a variation of that lift that you can choose while you iron out the weakness. The first rule of choosing your assistance moves is to identify the weakness in the main lift and work to strengthen that. Then there are assistance moves to build hypertrophy and then assistance moves to develop conditioning and work capacity as required.

How flexible are assistance moves?

I never speak in absolutes. It's never a case of 'always this' or 'never that'. In this system, in reality, there are two lower body strength sessions and two upper body strength sessions, so I can address the bench press twice a week, and the same for the overhead press, squat and deadlift.

As an example, assistance for the deadlift could very well be leg press and reverse hyperextensions. The leg press helps break the floor and the reverse hyperextension will help to build the spinal erectors and the glutes. You can't tell me that the extra leg strength from the leg press won't translate positively to the squat. You can't tell me that increased glute activation and spinal erector strength won't benefit the squat. So they complement each other. The assistance for deadlifts and deadlifting itself, will improve squatting.

On lower body day, assistance will always address trunk stability. They'll always address glutes, quads and hamstrings. Remember, we're also putting loaded carries into the workouts, so we could be doing farmer's walks and Zercher carries, both of which will have a positive effect on deadlifts and squats. It's all part of one big picture.

Would I have someone squat more than once a week? Absolutely. Would I have someone deadlift more than once a week? One hundred per cent. But that's based on the individual. For someone at my level, on squat day I may very well use trap bar deadlifts as an assistance move. On deadlift day I could use front squats as an assistance to my deadlift. So in essence I will deadlift twice a week and squat twice a week. But it all depends on what the individual requires and, more importantly, what they can tolerate. We could put together a workout that looks good on paper and makes perfect sense, but if the individual can't recover then it needs re-evaluating.

> 'What is a coach? We're problem-solvers – because you rarely get people who fit into the perfect template with zero issues'

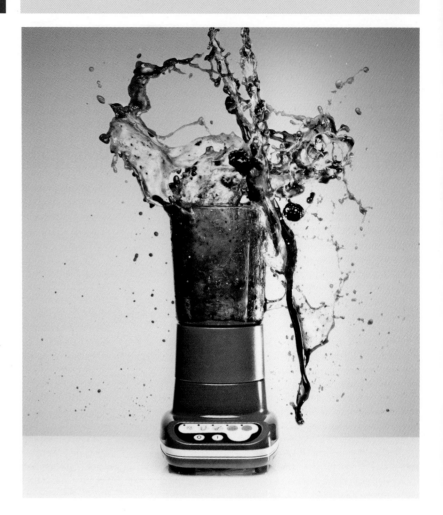

What do I do if progress stalls?

Despite the best efforts of a well planned programme, progress can stall from time to time. While this may be down to a small technical flaw on a certain movement or movements, most of the time I find it can be attributed to one of the following:

1. Sleep

Sleep is the ultimate performance enhancer. It is something everyone does, yet few ever truly appreciate or optimise. I took it for granted for a long time, not only as a competitive athlete, but also as a fledgling business owner. Seven hours minimum per night is a rule I instil in all my clients. *Why We Sleep* by the neuroscientist Professor Matthew Walker was a game-changer for me. I strongly recommend you check that out.

2. Application

Ask yourself honestly: just how hard do you train in your sessions? Do you give everything to every single set, rep and exercise? Are you the hardest worker in your gym right now? In my experience most people don't and aren't. Any programme, the better ones included, is only ever as good as how it is applied. You have to train very hard indeed in order to achieve results. Just remember it is how hard you train on each and every set and rep that counts, not how many sets and reps you do. Intensity is key!

3. Nutrition

Strength training requires very specific nutrition. In my experience that is nutrition that optimises gut health, fuels and sustains frequent demanding workouts, and maximises recovery between said workouts. If you cut corners here it will show in the gym. Underfuelled and undernourished lifters progress more slowly and pick up more injuries and colds than those who are on point.

4. Recovery

Training as intensely as I advocate takes a toll not just on your muscles, but on your nervous system too. Simply put, it is one big stress. Therefore, the harder you train, the harder you must recover. I've never seen a case of true overtraining.

I see cases of under-recovering daily. These are my go-to methods for those following a strength programme:

- Sleep a minimum of 7 hours nightly – longer is better
- Daily mobility, which includes walking and being active
- Epsom Salts bath daily (300-500g/bath)
- Sauna (every other day, minimum 20 minutes)
- Soft tissue therapy (ideally weekly, at least monthly)

The more aggressive you are with your recovery, the more productive your strength sessions can be. Just don't forget to train hard enough to warrant recovering from it.

When and how should I deload?

A deload sees you reduce the level of your training stress for a short period of time, typically, between seven and 10 days. For me programming a deload is just as important as programming training. They should be factored in strategically. In my experience scheduling a deload every four to six weeks works very well.

Exactly how you deload is both specific to you as an individual as well as your current training style and goal. I look to three separate types of deload for strength training as oulined in this book.

1. VOLUME DELOAD
I feel it is important to still handle heavy weights in order to keep your nervous system on point, so you can do a volume deload – one that will focus on a reduction in training volume. You can do so in one of the below ways:

A. Reduce reps per set
If on a normal training week your main lift workout prescribes 5 x 6 @ 100kg, a volume deload would see this reduce to 5 x 3 @ 100kg. You still lift the same weight (100kg) for the same amount of sets but reduce the reps by 50%.

The same goes for your assistance exercises which may be prescribed as 4 x 8-12. During the volume deload this would become 4 x 4-6. The weight on these exercises remains the same; all that changes are the reps per set. This is the option I use most frequently with my strength-focused clients.

B. Reduce sets per exercise
In this case exercises, weights and reps remain the same. Simply perform 2-3 fewer sets per exercise in order to decrease volume for a deload.

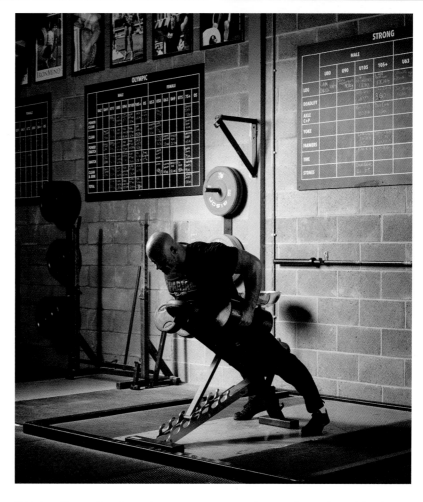

C. Reduce the number of exercises
This is my least preferred option. You can volume deload by keeping sets, reps and weights the same and dropping all exercises bar two – the main lift and a key assistance movement.

What all three of these options have in common is simple: you reduce your training volume (not intensity) by 40-50%.

2. INTENSITY DELOAD
Advocated by coaches like Chad Smith and Jim Wendler, intensity deloads typically involve performing your main lift at loads of 40-60% while reducing all assistance movements to 50% of their normal volume. I have found that those more experienced and accomplished in strength training, myself included, respond very well to a volume deload. An intensity deload works very well for those who are less experienced.

3. BUILD-UP WEEK
This is the method I factor into a mesocycle in which every fifth week marks the beginning of a new training phase. The first weeks see volume and intensity at their lowest and thus, in essence, they act as their own deload week of sorts. You can recover from the previous week's high intensity and volume while not overtaxing the CNS and still stay sharp in the process.

When programmed correctly this is a very effective method to sustain progress throughout a mesocycle while not burning out. While effective, it is certainly not one I use with beginners.